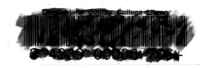

W9-CDU-193

THE AZTEC DIET

THE AZTEC DIET

Chia Power: The Superfood That Gets You Skinny and Keeps You Healthy

DR. BOB ARNOT

WILLIAM MORROW

An Imprint of HarperCollins*Publishers*

This book is written as a source of information only. The information contained in this book should by no means be considered a substitute for the advice of a qualified medical professional, who should always be consulted before beginning any new diet, exercise, or other health program.

All efforts have been made to ensure the accuracy of the information contained in this book as of the date published. The author and the publisher expressly disclaim responsibility for any adverse effects arising from the use or application of the information contained herein.

HarperCollins books may be purchased for educational, business, or sales promotional use. For information please write: Special Markets Department, HarperCollins Publishers, 10 East 53rd Street, New York, NY 10022.

FIRST EDITION

Designed by Richard Oriolo

Library of Congress Cataloging-in-Publication Data has been applied for.

ISBN 978-0-06-212405-0

13 14 15 16 17   DIX/RRD   10 9 8 7 6 5 4 3 2 1

Bobby and Hayden Arnot:

Dedicated to my two wonderful sons, Bobby and Hayden,

who have brought me so much joy and inspiration.

For their undying loyalty to their father. Not an hour goes by

that I don't think of them. Their hard work and diligence

are an endless source of inspiration to me.

Aztec Diet

[az-tek **dahy**-it]

noun

1. A three-phase diet, based on the foods of the Aztecs, that will achieve and maintain healthy weight and blood sugar levels.

CONTENTS

PHASE II

PHASE III

GLOSSARY

AZTEC FOODS

noun, pl.

1. Foods that fueled the ancient Aztec Empire. High in protein, low in carb load and inflammation. Examples: chia, quinoa, amaranth, beans, corn, fish, turkey, tomatoes.

CARB LOAD

noun

1. A food's capacity to raise blood sugar factored with the amount of carbohydrate in the food, expressed as a single number.

Synonyms: glucose load and glycemic load

CARB BOMB

noun

1. A carbohydrate that releases a large amount of sugar into the bloodstream.

2. Your new enemy.

CHIA

noun

1. "A plant, *Salvia hispanica*, native to central and southern Mexico and Guatemala: the seeds are used as food." *Dictionary.com. Salvia* derives from the Latin *salvare*: To feel well and healthy; health; heal.

2. Cornerstone of the ancient Aztec diet.

3. Key to successful weight loss, weight management, energy, and blood sugar regulation.

4. Your new best friend.

INFLAMMATION

noun

1. "*Pathology.* redness, swelling, pain, tenderness, heat, and disturbed function of an area of the body, especially as a reaction of tissues to injurious agents." *Dictionary.com.*

FLAME THROWER

noun

1. A highly inflammatory food. Flame throwers are leading contributors to obesity, diabetes, heart disease, and depression. They are high in saturated fat, high in omega-6 fatty acids, high in carb load, and low in omega-3 fatty acids. Examples: white flour, white rice, enriched spaghetti, white bread, and flour tortillas.

2. Your other new enemy.

SCORING FOODS

S coring foods is how we discovered that Aztec foods have the best nutrition profiles of the smorgasbord of foods available today, 500 years after the fall of the Aztec Empire.

Scoring systems are rapidly gaining popularity, so you may have seen some of them at the supermarket. Whole Foods Market uses the ANDI (Aggregate Nutrient Density Index) scale, which scores foods based on their nutrient contents on a scale from one to 1,000. CSPI (Center for Science in the Public Interest), a food organization I greatly admire and reported on for years, reveals not only a food's impact on your health, but the effect of its cultivation on the environment and even animal welfare.

We've pored through all the most important scientific databases to identify healthy foods for you, and throughout this book you will find tables that reference various criteria we have used to rate foods. The data in these tables come from sources such as the USDA's National Nutrient Database for Standard Reference, the most extensive source of nutrition data. You may find Whole Foods ANDI scale and Conde Nast's NutritionData website the most useful because they make it so easy to look up individual foods. If you'd like to know more about the scoring categories, you can read more in the descriptions that follow. You may also want to visit the following websites, which are excellent resources for determining the carb loads of your favorite foods.

- http://www.ncbi.nlm.nih.gov/pmc/articles/PMC2584181/bin/dc08-1239_index.html (University of Sydney tables)

- http://nutritiondata.self.com (Conde Nast's SELF NutritionData)

- http://www.mendosa.com/gilists.htm (a useful list of CLs for many common foods)

- http://www.health.harvard.edu/newsweek/Glycemic_index_and_glycemic_load_for_100_foods.htm (Harvard University)

SCORING CATEGORIES

ANDI:

The Whole Foods Market rating system tallies all nutritional elements to determine an overall score between one and 1,000. The higher the score the more nutritious the food. This system highlights the all-important micronutrient content in fruits, vegetables, beans, and grains.

CL:

Carb load, also known as glycemic load, is most helpful for grains, and will help you steer clear of carb bombs. CL measures the rise in blood sugar caused by a food based on the amount of carbohydrate in the food.

- The very best foods have CLs in the single digits.

- Foods with a CL of 10–20 are considered moderate.

- Stay away from carb bombs that have CLs of 20 or higher.

- Chia has a CL of just one.

If you're trying to lose weight quickly or get your blood sugar firmly under control, aim for a daily total CL of 50. The upper limit of what's considered healthy is 100.

Fullness:

Foods with high scores in this category will fill you up; low scores will leave you wanting. Hot dogs, for instance, have a very low fullness score, which is probably why people often go back for seconds and thirds at barbecues!

Inflammation:

High positive numbers in this scoring system mean that a food is an antioxidant with anti-inflammatory properties. Negative numbers indicate that a food causes inflammation in the body. Aim for a daily score of 50 or higher. Any food that scores –200 or lower qualifies as a flame thrower! Steer clear. Inflammation is highest in refined grains and lowest in vegetables.

Fat percentage:

In the meats section we list the percentage of total calories in each meat that is comprised of fat. This number quickly identifies the most efficient proteins, or those that give you the most amount of protein and fullness with the least amount of fat. A quick look at the table shows that turkey and chicken are highly efficient while hot dogs are not. There are also some cuts of beef that are quite lean.

Omega-6 and Omega-3s:

These numbers indicate quantity rather than a scoring system. Choose foods that have high amounts of omega-3s and avoid those with lots of omega-6s. For some foods we note the ratio of omega-6s to omega-3s. The highest omega-3s are found in fish and chia. The highest omega-6s are found in vegetable oils and certain nuts.

AAS (Amino Acid Score):

There are 9 essential amino acids, which are the building blocks of muscles and other tissues. AAS measures the number and type of amino acids in a food. The higher the score, the higher the quality of a protein. An AAS of 100 or higher signifies a complete protein. You may be surprised to learn that chia, quinoa, and black beans all rate higher than most cuts of meat.

Other nutrients:

We list quantities of relevant nutrients to help you select foods that are low in calories and high in protein and fiber. For instance, we have a table showing the amount of calcium found in dairy products and substitutes to be sure you're getting enough.

CHAPTER 1

THE AZTEC DIET AND THE MIRACLE SEED

Howare you?"

"Never better," I answer, every time I'm asked. I mean it. In all my years I've never felt better, looked leaner, worked more productively, or performed better at sports. Why? I've dropped the foods that have poisoned so many of us for so long and embraced the foods of the ancient Aztecs—foods that give me boundless energy, a bright mental attitude, and endless creativity. How is all this possible? With the Aztec Diet! By following the guidelines in this book, and the eating habits of a mighty ancient civilization, you will soon find yourself feeling the same.

The Aztec Diet will transform your body, health, mind, attitude, and life by harnessing the power of the ancient Aztec superfood chia, and eliminating the foods that wreak havoc on our systems: carb bombs (foods like bagels, pretzels, granola, pancakes, and enriched spaghetti, which jack up blood sugar and leave you ravenous when they plummet) and flame throwers (foods like white flour, white rice, and flour tortillas, which bring sky-high levels of inflammation into the body).

Two out of three Americans eat diets loaded with these dangerous foods. That means that you most likely eat foods every day that wreak havoc on blood sugar, weight, health, and mood! No wonder you've been having a hard time keeping your energy up while trying to diet! The blood of most people on a classic, carb-loaded Western diet has become a poisonous, angry stew of altered hormones and elevated blood fats, inflammation, cholesterol, and sugars. The carbs spike blood sugar to unmanageable highs; a nasty cycle ensues as the blood sugar level crashes, creating ravenous hunger for more carbs to boost blood sugar back up. This makes us feel fatigued and sluggish on a daily basis. Sound familiar? Eventually we get sick, suffering heart disease, stroke, cancer, diabetes, high blood pressure, Alzheimer's, and death.

The incredibly great news, though, is that this cycle can be broken quickly and easily. As simple as it sounds, you can eradicate these dangers by changing the foods you eat with the Aztec Diet. You do not have to be fatigued. You do not have to be overweight. A skinnier, more energetic, healthier, and happier you is possible.

In this book we'll teach you how to change the foods you eat by calling on one of the most successful civilizations in history. Eating the foods of the Aztecs, who for centuries dominated all of central Mexico, will:

- **Kill your cravings**

- **Brighten your mood**

- **Supercharge your energy**

- **Melt the pounds away**

You won't have to use raw willpower or endure gnawing hunger. The Aztec foods will do the job of losing weight for you.

If you struggle to manage a high carb load, feeling light-headed, shaky, lethargic, and starved when your blood sugar comes crashing down, the Aztec Diet is for you.

If you, like so many, have tried a million diets and still have trouble controlling your weight, the Aztec Diet is for you. Give your body a break. Give yourself a break. You haven't failed at dieting, the foods you eat have failed you, and your key to success is in the following pages.

Too good to be true? Not at all. In fact, we have centuries of proof that the Aztec diet works effectively:

- Aztec foods are the healthiest foods on the planet and fueled one of the most powerful empires in history. They include beans, corn, turkey, fish, vegetables, fruit, and super grains such as amaranth, bulgar, quinoa, and one that you may never have heard of but will change your life: chia. Substituting these foods for high-carb, high-sugar, high-fat foods will quickly render you the leanest, fittest, and most energetic you've ever been.

- AD foods are filling and taste great! The foods in this diet are packed with nutrients and can radically change your metabolism. Most so-called diet foods have little flavor and are only marginally healthier than the foods that make us fat. You don't have to sacrifice taste to lose weight.

- The AD is simple so you can sustain it anywhere, anytime without complicated meal plans, calorie counting, or prepared meals or bars. At the diet's most basic level, there is a simple morning smoothie and a few basic substitutions to your current diet. I lead a fast life on the run and have no time for complex shopping lists or food preparation. I prepare my breakfast smoothie, which is rich in every imaginable nutrient, in fewer than 60 seconds. Time is one of the biggest roadblocks to eating well, so one of the major breakthroughs of the AD is that it turns great food into fast food.

- Losing weight on the AD happens quickly and effectively, preventing the feelings of frustration or failure that cause people to abandon healthy eating. With a kick-start to your weight loss, you'll be incredibly pleased with your progress and much more likely to keep going.

- With Aztec foods at the core of your diet, you can reward yourself with treats so you don't feel deprived. You can splurge when you want and return to this core when you're tired, you've gained a few pounds, or you're just feeling unhealthy. You'll be amazed at how easily you can recover from weddings, holidays, and vacations. Now you can enjoy those events without the guilty dieter's mentality, knowing that returning to the Aztec foods will quickly get you back to fighting weight.

THE MIRACLE SEED

As a physician, author, fitness enthusiast, endurance athlete, and medical journalist, I've always had an eye out for the next big nutritional breakthrough. In working as a medical correspondent for *Dateline*, the *Today* show, the *NBC Nightly News*, *CBS This Morning*, and the *CBS Evening News*, I discovered that nutrition stories make the most interesting news because they are so immediately actionable and have such a big impact on our lives. I can tell you, however, that true breakthroughs don't happen often. Diet books, superfoods, and supplements offer new hope, then fizzle fast.

So, when a great friend, Lizzie Hinckley, said she had a miracle food product, I politely put her off. Lizzie's an amazing ski racer, sailor, and horsewoman. During winters in Stowe, Vermont, we'd ski downhills against each other. Side by side we'd hit 50 miles per hour racing to get to the bottom first. It was pure, terrifying exhilaration. In the summer we'd pit our endurance against each other on epic 70-mile bike rides. With a staggering power-to-weight ratio, Lizzie climbed like a gazelle, while I struggled to keep her in sight.

One day in late February 2010, after a downhill on Mount Mansfield's Hayride racing trail, Lizzie shared her secret. She dropped a shiny bag onto the backseat of my motorcycle. I left it out in the snow for days. She kept texting me: "Did you try it?" I finally took the bag off my prized Ducati racing bike, dusted off the snow, and went straight to the FDA nutrition label on the back of the package. No. Could it be true? *Five* grams of fiber in just 70 calories? The rest of the ingredient list read like a bestseller. I could hardly believe that so many nutrients could be packed into just one food.

I logged on to the Internet to read about chia. Gram for gram, it outperforms all of the world's healthiest foods. Chia has:

- 8 times more omega-3s than Atlantic farmed salmon, the most in any whole food

- 6 times more calcium than milk

- 3 times more iron than spinach

- 2 times more fiber than bran flakes

- 15 times more magnesium than broccoli

- 4 times more selenium than flax

I've always been a fan of supergrains. I eat whole-grain breads and the highest-fiber cereals; I love quinoa and amaranth, the golden grains of the Aztecs. But chia? I'd never heard of it. After a quick Google search I was mesmerized.

The chia story began in 2500 B.C., but the little seed later acquired its fame from the Aztec warriors. The Aztecs cultivated amazing foods that gave them the strength and energy to build one of civilization's great empires. One of those was a super seed called *chia.* Corn, chia, and beans were the Aztecs' three staple foods. But it was chia alone, which they called "the running food," that sustained Aztec warriors during their long journeys and frequent battles. When wounded in battle or on hunting expeditions, the Aztecs packed their wounds with this "miracle seed" to help fight infection. Chia was so fundamental to the Aztecs' success and beliefs that the Spanish burned the vast chia production fields as part of their campaign to destroy the Aztec civilization. This agricultural annihilation, the Europeans' superior fire power, and the diseases they carried proved too much for the Aztecs, who vanished into the mists of time.

After the Spanish defeated the Aztecs, chia grew wild in the American West and Mexico, but disappeared from large-scale agricultural production and was largely forgotten. That's why you may have heard of supergrains like quinoa or amaranth, but not chia. Native Americans grew and ate chia for hundreds of years after the Spanish destroyed the chia fields. These hardy warriors found that chia provided so much energy that they could run messages all the way from the Colorado River to the Pacific Ocean, or spend days hunting on foot with no more than chia to eat, often just two spoonfuls per day. They crossed deserts in extreme heat with little water or food, except chia. Edward Palmer, in his botanical travels over deserts and through Mexico, wrote in 1891 that chia was one of the "best relished and most nutritive foods." Today, superathletes use chia as a fuel for grueling long-distance bike races and professional sports.

Chia regained some popularity in the 1960s in California health food stores. Food scientist Dr. Al Bushway bought his first chia in 1978 and has studied it at the University of Maine in the Department of Food Science and Human Nutrition since the early

1980s. Agricultural production only began to scale up again in 2005. It wasn't until the last few years that a serious effort was put into scientific study of chia's benefits, and not until the spring of 2010 that its remarkable effect on weight loss began to emerge. Awareness of the little seeds got a big boost in 2009 with the publication of Christopher McDougall's book, *Born to Run*, which put most endurance athletes in awe of the Tarahumara Indians from Mexico's Copper Canyon. They ran staggering distances, up to 200 miles in one session, with the ease that most of us use to cross our living rooms, eating little but chia.

I was sold based on the nutritional benefits but dreaded the taste test. I poured ground chia onto my cereal. No taste at all! Then I tried it in water. The ground seeds expanded and softened in the liquid but, again, no real taste. In almond milk, the ground chia added a pleasant texture. It is such a great mixer that it was easy to incorporate into my diet. For a similar nutrient value I could eat ten bowls of brussels sprouts, cauliflower, spinach, or broccoli—or four scoops of chia. What a no-brainer! What an incredibly easy way to pack in nutrients and lose weight without consuming massive amounts of vegetables!

Chia is easy to add to your diet and needs little preparation. If you buy whole seeds you should grind them in a coffee-bean or other grinder, as whole seeds tend to pass through the digestive system, and eat them right away so they don't go rancid. We recommend buying ground or micro-sliced chia, the best of which won't go rancid and can be added directly to foods and drinks, sprinkled and stirred right in. Chia is most effective when hydrated, so adding it to liquids (especially smoothies!) is the best way to go. Consider investing in a high-speed blender such as a Vitamix to make your smoothies. For more on these, see page 34.

I turned next to my own nutritional challenge. I had been stuck at 208 pounds for five years and was as heavy as 225 when my wife was pregnant with our first son. No matter how hard I tried, no matter how much I starved myself or how much I exercised, the best I could do was to hit 203, only to bounce back up to 208. I'd tried all the diets: Atkins, South Beach, Zone, you name it. Part of the problem was that I was pretty fit and just couldn't lose those last 15 pounds. I knew that if I could stop eating in the late afternoon I could lose a pound per day with all the exercise I do, but I just couldn't stand the brain-drain from low blood sugar, and the hunger pangs would drive me to raid the fridge in the evenings. Chia changed everything. I ate a scoop at 3:00 P.M. At midnight I had eaten nothing else. How could it be?

- No hunger pangs

- No loss of brain energy

- No shaky feeling of low blood sugar

I was stunned. Then I started to look at the scale. Every day that I wanted to, I lost a pound. In fact, I had to hold myself back from losing too much weight too quickly. When I added up the calories, I was eating only 800 a day. Too little. I had to back off the chia so I'd lose weight more slowly. But the scale still amazed me: 204, 203, 202, 201, 200. Two hundred? I hadn't been there in twenty years. Then my weight started to plummet: 198, 196, 194, 192. I was a different person metabolically and physically. As an avid amateur bike racer, I had never raced faster. I was beating kids in their twenties. I could do things like lunges, which I hadn't done since junior high! I felt fantastic. At 188 pounds I was healthy and lean and stunned at the effectiveness of chia.

Chia didn't only help me drop pounds. It gave me an enormous sense of calm and quiet energy. It allowed me to work long hours each day and preserve intense energy for killer workouts on cross-country skis, downhill racing skis, bikes, and paddleboards. It also gave me self-control. Two years ago I approached dinner buffets like a vacuum cleaner. Now I walk into dinners fearlessly, knowing that I can pick at them like a fussy kid.

Eager to share chia's incredible benefits, I created a diet with this grain as its cornerstone. It may seem odd to focus a diet on a single food, but chia is so nutritious and so filling that it's an unparalleled powerhouse. Chia serves as a gateway food, demonstrating just how powerful one food can be, then lures dieters into making other spectacular choices.

Phase One of the Aztec Diet, which consists of three chia smoothies a day plus snacks, launches a total metabolic breakthrough.

In Phase Two, you can accelerate your weight loss by adding a well-chosen lunch to fuel your transformed metabolism.

Phase Three returns to regular meals consisting of the healthiest premium foods on earth, primarily foods of the Aztecs.

Finally, there is advice for recovery when (not if) you give in to the urge to splurge. We all do it. To expect it and have a plan for recovery makes all the difference. I can hardly wait to go back on the Aztec Diet after big dietary indulgences. I recently came back from a trip to the Middle East and Africa the heaviest I'd been since first beginning the Aztec Diet. I was up to 203.8 pounds by the time I got home, but within a week I was at 198.2 pounds. Within three weeks I was back at 189 pounds.

The Aztec Diet is the culmination of my lifelong, worldwide search for the very best foods and the most effective diet of all time. We've done the homework for you. We've ranked foods according to their carb loads (the lower the better!) and other important nutritional information; we offer meal suggestions, recipes, and strategies for sound sleep, exercise, and coping with tough situations. This time, losing weight will be easy, and it will stay off!

HOW TO USE THIS BOOK:

Most of you reading this book have weight to lose. All of you probably suffer from fatigue and could use a big boost in energy. You fight cravings for foods that only make matters worse. Whether you realize it or not, your bodies suffer from unnecessary inflammation, causing pain and threatening illness.

Use this book to feel better. The next chapter will explain in detail why the Aztec Diet works. After that, the book will guide you through losing weight, eliminating cravings, calming inflammation, increasing energy, and learning healthy eating habits you can use for the rest of your life.

Part I will help you change your metabolism and guide you through fast, effective weight loss with a diet of three chia smoothies each day.

Part II will replace the midday smoothie with a carefully chosen lunch to propel you past the classic dieters' plateau. You'll fuel your body for productive afternoons, making exercise a true pleasure.

Part III is your guide for making smart, nutritious food choices for the rest of your life. You'll learn how to select foods, gather new recipes, and garner tips on sleeping well and incorporating exercise into your life.

Much more than a weight-loss plan, this book will teach you how to feel the best you ever have in your life.

CHAPTER 2

WHY THE AZTEC DIET WORKS

On most diets you're running on empty with brain-searing hunger, stretching the upper limits of self-control. Acid churns in your stomach as digestive enzymes gush into your intestines after each tiny morsel. You're famished within minutes after eating. You watch time tick by, counting down until your next meal, and each minute seems like an hour. On the Aztec Diet, you'll feel better than you ever believed you could. This is because the AD accomplishes five incredibly powerful tasks:

1. **Fills you up**

2. **Dumps the carb bombs**

3. **Douses the fire inside**

4. **Pours on the supernutrients**

5. **Makes your brain feel great**

Let's take a look at why these things are so important and how they work to help your weight plummet.

1. FILL 'ER UP!

The first benefit of the AD is that you stay full so you don't have to suffer. Here's how it works.

Food Expansion Within the Stomach

The AD gives you a natural way of decreasing the available space for more food in your stomach, which signals to your brain that your stomach is full, so you stop eating. Stomach bypass surgery for the severely overweight has become the most successful weight-loss measure on record. Part of that procedure severely shrinks the stomach so it can't hold a lot of food. At the cutting edge of medical research, doctors are implanting mechanical devices in the stomach that expand to fill it up and make the patient feel full. Chia mimics these surgical successes naturally by expanding up to seven times its size in your stomach, drastically decreasing the space available for food and making you feel full. The AD is the first diet to take full advantage of this principle.

Food Volume: Eat More to Weigh Less

The AD gives you a large volume of food to keep you full. Most diets err by giving you too little food, often food that is densely packed with calories. I can't believe the "diet" dinners I see in the frozen foods section of the supermarket. Pancakes. Pizza. Yikes! Sure, the portions are small and the calories are few, but let's be honest. Just how long would you last after eating a small wedge of frozen pizza before wanting to dive into something else? If you eat the right foods, you can eat them until you're sated.

The gratifying success story of the Hawaiian Diet exemplifies the eat-more-to-weigh-less concept better than any other. In the 1990s native Hawaiians had the worst health-care statistics of any population in the United States. Obesity and diabetes were so prevalent they endangered an entire culture. Dr. Terri Shintani, who trained at the Harvard School of Public Health, made a basic appeal to Hawaiians: return to your cultural and spiritual values by embracing the foods of your ancestors.

According to Hawaiian lore, Wakea, Father Heaven, bore a son named Haloa with Daughter of Earth. Born prematurely and shaped like a bulb, the child died and was buried at one corner of the house. The couple's second-born was a strong, healthy son, also named Haloa, who became the ancestor of all the Hawaiian people. He was to respect and care for his elder brother, who would come to be known as taro, the root of life. Taro, in turn, would nourish Haloa and all his descendants. Taro has remarkable health benefits, including weight-loss properties and a carb load of only 2. By returning to taro and other traditional foods, Hawaiians could triple the volume of food they ate, yet lose vast amounts of weight, because their foods were dense in nutrients, not calories.

Soon it was clear that this worked. For a CBS broadcast, I profiled a man known as "Big Ed." Ed was really big, weighing 425 pounds. His blood sugar soared to 800, his cholesterol reached 285, and he required 80 units of insulin a day. Dr. Shintani showed Big Ed pictures of his ancestors, who were tall, lean, muscular people standing alongside monster surf boards. Rather than lecture Big Ed on the dangers of fast foods, Shintani encouraged him to embrace the values of his Hawaiian heritage. Ed did so with vigor. Best of all, he didn't have to starve; he was told to eat as much as he wanted. Since native Hawaiian foods are high in fiber and low in calories and carb load, he was so satiated that he couldn't finish his meals. We later demonstrated this striking difference in food volume for a *Dateline NBC* show on the Hawaiian Diet. We showed two plates side by side, one bearing 1¾ pounds of fast food, the other piled with 4¼ pounds of traditional Hawaiian foods. While the Hawaiian plate contained much more food, it had far fewer calories and much less cholesterol, fat, and sugar.

When we returned to Oahu, Big Ed had lost 150 pounds, his blood sugar and cholesterol were within the normal range, and he had stopped taking insulin. The diet was so successful that the governor and his cabinet also embraced it with remarkable success. I fell in love with the concept. I found Shintani a publisher for the book he'd written about the diet and wrote its foreword. What I found so alluring about Shintani's approach was its contrast to the stern and widely ignored public health warnings. By imploring people to embrace their culture, heritage, and spiritual values, the Hawaiian Diet proved an incredible success. Researchers worldwide are finding that traditional plant foods of indigenous cultures can benefit all of us. Look into your own ethnic background for foods that made your ancestors lean and healthy, and embrace them. Or go straight for the most powerful foods of all: Aztec foods.

Slowed Stomach Emptying

Chia breaks down slowly so it slows stomach emptying naturally, keeping you full far longer than other foods do. People on the Aztec Diet routinely tell me that hours go by without their ever thinking about eating. This is especially useful in the late morning, midafternoon, and evening, when we're most tempted to overeat. With chia on board you'll find that temptation evaporates. New mechanical devices are attempting to slow stomach emptying.[1] You can delay emptying in a completely natural way with chia.

Slowed Absorption

Chia is absorbed more slowly from the small intestine into your bloodstream than most Western foods so you remain satisfied hours longer than after your usual meals. This also means that you'll have a smoother, slower rise of sugars and fats in the blood after meals. Since rapidly falling blood sugar makes us ravenously hungry, the foods of the AD will take away the enormous craving that so many of us have developed for sugar. Even when you indulge in sweet treats, the AD will slow the absorption of that sugar to blunt its effect.

WHERE'S THE EVIDENCE?[2]

A classic study by Dr. Vladimir Vuksan, published in the *European Journal of Clinical Nutrition*, showed that high doses of chia (*Salvia hispanica L.*) decreased appetite 60 minutes, 90 minutes, and 120 minutes after eating. This also decreased the usual rise in blood sugar that follows a meal rich in carbohydrates. This decrease in blood sugar after AD meals may also explain the improvement in blood pressure, coagulation, and inflammation levels. Chia does that by helping you slash your carb load, as we'll see next.[3]

2. DUMP THE CARB BOMBS!

Being full makes it much easier to shed excess sugar. An enormous amount of the carbohydrate we eat is excess sugar and is just plain wasted. Our blood sugar levels spike as our bodies look for an emergency location to store the vast amounts of sugar we pour into our stomachs. Where does it go? You guessed it. That storage depot is FAT. The average American eats more carbs than our systems were designed to handle at any one meal and far more than our bodies have been able to adapt to in the mere century since sugars and refined foods became widely available. Constant spikes in blood sugar wear out the body's ability to handle sugar. Insulin is used by most of the body's cells to absorb glucose from the blood for use as fuel and for storage. As the pancreas struggles to produce more and more insulin, it finally just gives up. The result is diabetes. Without enough insulin, we quickly get sick.

A critically important point to take away from this book is that a sharp rise and subsequent fall in blood sugar is one of the greatest causes of hunger. By eating foods that don't spike your blood sugar, you'll prevent one of the most vexing problems in the American diet. Most people know that sweets will spike their blood sugar (and pile on the pounds!), but most of the grains we eat also contain too many sugars for the body to handle at one time. Complex carbohydrates with high carb loads are the real villains in our diets. They look like perfectly innocent foods, but when they land in the stomach they unload a huge packet of sugar that overwhelms the body's ability to handle it. Think of these carbs that appear moderate—bagels, bread, rice cakes, nonfat fruit yogurt, and pancakes—as carb bombs. Food grenades! Tossing one into the stomach spews damage in every direction. The excess sugar stresses every aspect of our bodies and damages our blood vessels and internal organs.

The Mighty River

Here's another analogy. Picture a mighty river like the Mississippi. The river has a maximum amount of water it can handle. When massive rainfall exceeds that amount, the river overflows its banks, destroying everything in its wake: bridges, schools, homes, cars, levees, and crops. The extra water does nothing to improve the flow of water downstream or the function of the river. It's only destructive. The same is true of excess sugar in our bloodstreams. The sugar overflows its banks like a mighty river, wreaking havoc in our bodies. We feel momentarily good as our blood sugar spikes and then dreadful as it falls. In fact our brains panic. Because the brain's main fuel is sugar, when it senses a drop we feel famished and race to eat even more sugar.

Smooth Blood Sugar Levels

AD meals are designed with just the right amount and quality of carbohydrates for our bodies to handle smoothly so our blood sugar levels don't spike. This curtails the tremendous excesses that have caused the largest obesity epidemic in history. How fast does the transition to a smoother blood sugar level take? It happens literally in the span of a single meal. That is the enormous metabolic breakthrough of the AD. The lean, nutrient-dense foods of the AD don't spill any sugar. Carb bombs are replaced by stunning grains that will change your life forever. With no more carb bombs, there are no blood sugar spikes, no cravings, and no weight gain. The body is primed to shed weight.

Carb Load (CL)

This number will be the key to your new eating habits. Each carbohydrate can be measured for its ability to raise blood sugar levels. The result is scored as a single number we call *carb load* (scientifically referred to as *glucose load*). Low CLs are 1–10, moderate 10–20, and over 20 is considered high. A food with a high number, like white bread, will cause your blood sugar to soar and then crash.

You might find online sites that list the glycemic index of foods; please note that this is not the same as carb load or glucose load, though they are related. The glycemic index measures the speed at which a carb releases glucose into the bloodstream. Carb or glucose load measures both the speed of glucose release and the amount of carbohydrate in the food for a more complete picture. For you mathematical types, the formula looks like this:

CL = GI x the amount of carbohydrate in a 100-gram serving

High carb load puts both men and women at greater risk for obesity and diabetes, according to pioneering research conducted over the last fifteen years by the Harvard School of Public Health. (Also a major risk factor, researchers found, is low cereal fiber consumption.) Harvard's legendary professor Walter Willett concluded that the vast majority of diabetes can be *prevented*. The National Institutes of Health's analysis reinforces his finding, asserting that as much as 80 percent of type II diabetes can be prevented.

Pay attention to your overall carb load per meal and per day. Adding a 12-ounce Coke to a lunch of black bean salad will give you a modest rise in blood sugar, but if you consume a bowl of spaghetti, two rolls, and a slice of pizza, you'll suffer a major spike in blood sugar. A small square of chocolate causes only a small rise in blood sugar, whereas a half loaf of white bread causes it to soar. If you eat cereal for breakfast, crackers for snack, a sandwich for lunch, and pasta for dinner, your overall carb load for the day will be sky high. In this book you'll find tables listing carb loads for many foods. The scores vary slightly across different databases but they're good indicators of what a food will do to your blood sugar. Feel free to look up foods yourself using the links on page xv. Get to know these numbers well; they're your new best friends!

Let's have a look at three levels of carb loads: 0–10, 11–20, and 21+:

HEALTHY CARB LOAD	0–10
Corn tortilla, 2	10
Sprouted wheat bread, 2 slices	10
Honey, 1 tablespoon	10
Whole wheat crackers (Triscuit), 1 ounce	10
Microwave popcorn, low-fat, 1 ounce	10
Trail mix, 1.5 ounces	10
Quinoa, ½ cup cooked	9
Rye crackers (Wasa), 1 ounce	9
Greek yogurt (Fage, 0%)	8
Whole wheat pasta, ½ cup cooked	7.5
Kellogg's Special K Protein Plus, ¾ cup	5
Quaker Puffed Wheat, 1¼ cups	7
Bulgur, ½ cup cooked	6
Edamame, 1 cup	6
Chia, 2 ounces	2
Wheat bran, ½ cup	2
Celery, 2 stalks	2

LIGHT CARB LOAD	11–20
Kellogg's low-fat granola bar, 1	18
Rice milk, enriched original, 250 ml	17
Kashi GOLEAN Crunch, 1 cup	17
Cornflakes, 1 cup	17
Fruit leather, 1 ounce	17
Nature's Path Optimum Slim 1 cup	16
Pancake, 1 6"	15
Sweet potato, 1 large baked	15
Uncle Sam Cereal, 1 cup	15
Pretzels, 1 ounce	15
Baked tortilla chips, 1 ounce	15
Oatmeal, regular, cooked, 1 cup	14

CARB BOMBS	21+
Muesli, 1 cup	41
Plain bagel, 1 large	33
Hard pretzels, 10 twists	32
Homemade granola, 1 cup	31
Chocolate milkshake, 10 ounces	31
PowerBar, 1	29
Grapenuts, ½ cup	28
Raisin bran, 1 cup	26
Nonfat fruit yogurt, 1 cup	24
Spaghetti, enriched, 1 cup	23

CARB OVERLOAD, THE SCOURGE OF HUNTER-GATHERERS

The devastating effects of carb overload are best illustrated by the plight of hunter-gatherers who shifted suddenly to carb-heavy Western diets. In the 1960s geneticist James Neel developed a theory that a genetic adaptation allowed hunter-gatherers to store fat and calories with great efficiency so they could survive between kills and during times of famine. This "thrifty gene" enabled the survival of the Aztecs, Native Americans, indigenous Hawaiians, New Zealand's Maori, Arabia's bedouins, Canadian aborigines, and countless others whose meals were found sporadically and at long intervals. When they encountered the modern Western lifestyle and diet, these groups suffered the greatest weight gain in history and a savage epidemic of diabetes. Famine was no longer a problem. Tribes no longer had to wait for a kill to eat. The thrifty gene that had once allowed their survival became a terrible handicap when hunter-gatherers encountered Anglo foods that contained far more sugar and fat than their bodies could handle. Virtually all of these traditional peoples now suffer from punishing levels of obesity and diabetes.

The story of the Pima Indians best illustrates this tragic turn and the devastating power of high carb loads. The Pima came to North America across the land bridge roughly 34,000 years ago. With the whole continent at their disposal they chose to settle in the great Sonoran Desert with its scorching summer temperatures because, instinctively, they found that it grew the food that made them healthiest. Many crops contained a "sticky substance," or soluble fiber, which satiated them and allowed them to eat few calories while still maintaining a vigorous lifestyle.

The Pima thrived until Anglo settlers arrived, took their best land, and diverted the Gila River, disrupting a 2,000-year-old system of irrigation and agriculture. Beginning in the 1850s the Pima were increasingly constrained. Eventually, placed on a flour and lard diet of U.S. rations, the Pima rapidly gained weight. Their diet changed from high fiber and low fat (15 percent) to low fiber and high fat (40 percent). Now 95 percent of Pima age 35 and older are severely overweight. Half of them have type II diabetes, compared to one in 25 people in the general U.S. population. Amputations are so prevalent that children believe them to be standard treatment for diabetes. The obesity and diabetes lead to other afflictions, such as blindness, kidney failure, heart disease, hypertension, liver cirrhosis, and tooth decay.

I traveled to the Sierra Madre mountains of Mexico to visit another population of Pima. These people were rail thin with boundless energy. I met a 106-year-old man with whom I chatted long into the night. These Pima have very little diabetes, one-third less than the American population. Their diet? Beans, corn tortillas, salads, and peaches. While visiting them and sharing their foods I had boundless energy. Make a mental image of the two Pima populations and see what the right—and wrong—foods can do to you.

3. DOUSE THE FIRE INSIDE

You can bet that every overweight person you see is ablaze inside with raging inflammation. Research from Harvard's School of Public Health's Department of Nutrition shows that many foods that make us fat also pour inflammation into our bodies—every time we eat them, meal after meal, snack after snack. This makes the heart, lungs, brain, and other organs an angry, inflamed mess. A view inside inflamed coronary arteries is like looking at a bad case of acne: bright red artery walls with big yellow pimples ready to pop. Unlike most diets, the AD ranks foods based on inflammation so you can avoid the ones that are toxic.

FOOD	INFLAMMATION
White flour, 1 cup	−421
Hard pretzels, 10 twists	−229
Flour tortilla, 12"	−206
White rice, 1 cup	−153
Spaghetti (white flour), 1 cup	−122
Cornflakes, 1 cup	−100
Pancake, 1 6" pancake	−106
White bread, 1 slice	−53
Total	−1,390

We like to call the most inflammatory foods *flame throwers*. By contrast, AD foods can douse the fires of inflammation because they are packed with powerful antioxidants. In the very first hour of your new diet you began to soothe the inflammation in your body. If you tally your AD foods for the day, your antioxidant (inflammation) score should be 50 or higher. Inflammatory diets score negative 1,300 or worse. Individually the examples above are not the worst foods, but the effect of the daily total is staggering. Stay away from those flame throwers!

Here are examples of anti-inflammatory foods with *positive* scores. The higher the number, the better.

FOOD	ANTI-INFLAMMATION
Wild Pacific salmon, 3 ounces	582
Atlantic mackerel, 3 ounces	510
Spinach, 1 cup cooked	466
Canned anchovies, 1 can	461
Kale, 1 cup cooked	439
Collards, 1 cup cooked	379
Brazil nuts, 1 ounce	175
Flaxseed oil, 1 tablespoon	142
Macadamia nuts, 1 ounce	133
Guava, 1 cup	131
Cantaloupe, 1 cup	76
Pineapple, 1 cup	65
Strawberries, 1 cup	28

4. POUR ON THE SUPERNUTRIENTS

Ring Dings, Twinkies, french fries . . . I've snacked on junk for years, and I know how quickly it washes through you. You pull into a drive-through and pick up a cheeseburger and fries. After fifty miles on the highway, you're ready for another! Ever wonder why you continue to crave food when you feel full? It's because you didn't get all the nutrients you need. You're missing what we call *micronutrients*—minerals, vitamins, and antioxidants. Your body is on the hunt for these specific nutrients, and you'll remain hungry until your appetite for them has been satisfied. Millions of Americans eat many more fat and carbohydrate calories than they need because they're not getting the micronutrients they should. Research shows that 92 percent of Americans are lacking in one or more of the essential vitamins or minerals.

In a two-year study at Penn State, 7,500 people ate a diet that contained foods high in micronutrients (vitamins A, B$_6$, C, folate, iron, calcium, and potassium) but low in caloric density. The researchers found that the subjects drank fewer caloric carbonated beverages, consumed less fat, and ate fewer calories. Here's what they said:

> "*A high-micronutrient-density diet mitigates the unpleasant aspects of the experience of hunger even though it is lower in calories.* Hunger is one of the major impediments to successful weight loss. Our findings suggest that it is not simply the caloric content, but more importantly, the micronutrient density of a diet that influences the experience of hunger." They conclude that a high-nutrient-density diet can lead to weight loss and improved health.

The AD is brimming with nutrients, not calories. Satisfying that hunger for micronutrients will pave the way for truly sustainable weight loss and can also diminish disease. A 2010 study of flavonoid intakes, for example, found that high anthocyanin levels increased good-cholesterol levels.[4] Participants with the highest anthocyanin intake (predominantly from blueberries and strawberries) had an 8 percent reduction in risk of hypertension.[5] A powerful superfruit, blueberries are one of the AD's top ten fruits.

You don't have to take my word that Aztec foods contain staggering amounts of nutrients; one number says it all. Whole Foods Market's Aggregate Nutrient Density Index (ANDI) rates foods' nutrient content to guide consumers toward healthy choices. Add up the ANDI scores for a chia smoothie and you're over 3,000. The ANDI score for a hamburger, fries, and milkshake? It's only 70! We'll use ANDI throughout this book to compare foods.

You already know you should cut bad foods out of your diet, but the AD helps you add good things. Nutrients will make your mood soar and your waistline shrink. You'll feel great, and the numbers on your next blood test will further prove the point. Nearly all of our Aztec dieters saw their cholesterol, inflammation, and blood sugar levels plummet.

5. MAKE YOUR BRAIN FEEL GREAT

Your brain operates through a system of more than a trillion neurons that carry signals from one part of the brain to another. Think of those neurons as wires. If wires are old and tired with frayed casing, they conduct electricity poorly and at slow speeds. The latest efforts in neuroscience are aimed at improving the quality of the neuron, each one of which may have 10,000 connections! AD foods that are high in omega-3 fatty acids and a supplement we recommend called SAMe vastly improve the quality of the neuron, making it far more plastic with improved transmission. (See the "Supplements" section in the Appendix for high-quality brands of SAMe.) Such foods can even facilitate higher production of the neurotransmitters that allow one neuron to activate the next more readily. I describe this benefit as just plain feeling smarter. Complex projects suddenly seem simpler. The AD will unleash tremendous mental energy you may never have known you had. You'll wow yourself and your boss by working longer and better than ever. When I wake up, I swear I'm the clearest, smartest, and hardest working of my whole life. I find work a great pleasure and difficult tasks easy to perform.

REVIEW

This chapter may have seemed like complicated science, but the bottom line is simple. Keep your carb and inflammatory load low. The AD does the work for you, with meticulously constructed, delicious, filling meals. After your very first low-carb-load meal, your metabolism will start to change. Your blood sugar level will smooth out. The strain on your body will ease as you won't have to produce as much insulin. You'll feel calmer and more energetic. I notice the effects even today. I'll return from a business trip full of airline meals, fast foods, and dreadful dinners feeling old and haggard. The next morning, after my first chia smoothie, a sense of tremendous calm washes over me and my mental energy soars.

So, to review, just remember the five key principles: fill 'er up, dump the carb bombs, douse the fire inside, pour on the supernutrients, and make your brain feel great. Then the weight will start dropping. My friends and patients say this is the easiest weight loss they've ever experienced. And it's weight that stays off!

PHASE I

CHAPTER 3

PHASE I: THE CHIA CHALLENGE

THE PLAN: THREE CHIA SMOOTHIES A DAY

Phase One of the Aztec Diet is an aggressive program that will jump-start your weight loss faster than any diet you've tried. Like a cleanse, it gives you a break from all that is unhealthy. Unlike most cleanses, however, it supplies all the nutrients you need, keeping you full and energetic while you shed pounds at an incredible rate.

Chia is the heart of Phase One, and the best way to incorporate chia into your diet is through smoothies. During Phase One your daily menu couldn't be more simple. You'll drink three thick smoothies, which consist of a base, mixer, fruits and veggies, and, of course, chia, sipping them over a couple of hours. Snacks are permitted in the afternoon and evening, and you'll find a list of recommended ones at the end of this chapter. I have followed this diet myself, and every other diet I've tried comes in a distant second at best.

Usually, weight loss takes a very long time; that's because most plans introduce only modest changes in diet. When it takes so long to feel any results, many of us are discouraged from starting a diet or sticking with it. By contrast, the changes in Phase One of the AD, which we like to call the Chia Challenge, are so incredibly fast and effective that they constitute a total metabolic breakthrough.

Whether you're significantly overweight or simply want to feel better, stay on Phase One for two weeks. This will bring about profound improvements in your metabolism. If you need to lose 20 pounds or more and you're doing well, you can stick with it even longer. Participants in our Chia Challenge trial lost ½ to 1 pound per day, and some kept at it for 30 days, losing 30 pounds and more.

So many of us have been paralyzed by all the confusing, conflicting advice circulating on what we should do with our diets. The beauty of this chia smoothie is that it gives you *one actionable step* to vastly improve your diet and your health. It is important to *replace* your normal diet with the chia smoothie rather than add it to what you already eat. Because the smoothie will eliminate most of your carb and inflammatory load, it will make you feel dramatically better. That said, smoothie diets are not for everyone. I urge you to try it for at least one full day to see how good you feel. If it's not for you, don't return to your old eating habits! Instead, move on to Phase Three of the Aztec Diet, which is an incredibly healthy way to eat for the rest of your life.

SIMPLE AND FAST, THE CHIA CHALLENGE IS A 2-MINUTE, 2-DAY, 2-WEEK, 2-MONTH WONDER:

- In 2 minutes you can make the most nutritious meal on the planet.

- In 2 days your insulin and blood sugar levels will even out; you'll be down a few pounds; and your cholesterol, blood pressure, and inflammation will start to fall.

- In 2 weeks your metabolism will be totally recalibrated. Your LDL (bad cholesterol), triglycerides, and fasting blood sugar and weight will drop significantly if your results are anything like our challenge participants'. You'll be primed for exercise; you'll feel more energetic and you'll sleep more soundly.

■ In 2 months, having completed the Chia Challenge as well as Phase Two, you'll move on to the maintenance phase of the Aztec Diet as a different person physically, emotionally, and mentally. Svelte, healthy, and happy!

PHASE ONE

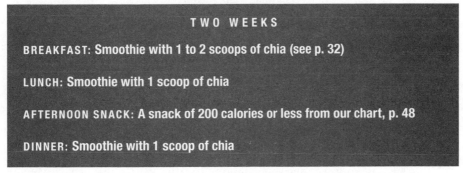

TWO WEEKS

BREAKFAST: Smoothie with 1 to 2 scoops of chia (see p. 32)

LUNCH: Smoothie with 1 scoop of chia

AFTERNOON SNACK: A snack of 200 calories or less from our chart, p. 48

DINNER: Smoothie with 1 scoop of chia

A study in the *American Journal of Clinical Nutrition* shows that favorable changes in the body's ability to handle blood sugar can occur in just three days. The catalyst for change in the study was simple. Subjects were fed a breakfast with a low carb load.

WARNING: (You won't find this in other diet books!) The AD is so effective that I had absolutely no hunger at all. I could easily drop to 800 calories a day, and that was just too little. Try to stick with the U.S. government weight-loss recommendations of 1 to 2 pounds a week. We want to encourage responsible weight loss. If you feel you're losing too fast, move on to Phase Two, which adds in lunch. If your weight is really plummeting, please talk to your doctor.

BEFORE YOU BEGIN

There aren't many barriers to beginning the AD. You could read this today, shop tonight, and start tomorrow. However, I do suggest some helpful first steps. These aren't required but will add to your resolve in moments of weakness and serve as proof of all the improvements you're making. If you have only 5 to 10 pounds to lose, don't worry about taking these steps. Jump right in!

As we tell all our dieters, please check with your doctor before starting a new program.

PICTURE PERFECT

Before you start, have a friend take photos of you. These are great to look back on because you'll soon change! Turn the camera vertically so you get a long, full-body shot. Measure the distance between you and the camera; aim for about 8 feet. Turn so that your left shoulder is facing the photographer and you are looking over it at him or her. Don't suck in your tummy. Just stand naturally. With a little space above your head and below your feet, you should fill most of the frame. Reshoot after two months using the same camera, lens, and zoom setting for an accurate comparison.

TAKE THE SURVEY

People are always stunned by how much better they feel after losing weight on the AD, and there are many solid medical reasons for this. To document improvements in mood, sleep, and other areas, fill out the Symptoms Questionnaire in the Appendix prior to starting the challenge. Retake it every fifteen days to see what's changed. You'll be amazed and very pleased.

WEIGH IN

Okay, this is where I differ from most diet experts. I am a firm believer in getting on the scale every day. You'll get a thrill every time another pound comes off. Even more important, daily weigh-ins show you how fast you can correct your course after an indulgent spell!

Directions

Weigh yourself just after you get up, after you've relieved yourself, and before you eat or drink anything. You should be buck naked. Weigh yourself at the same time every morning. I like a digital scale for its precision. Buy a high-quality one such as HoMedics. There's nothing more frustrating than seeing weight changes that are errors in the scale!

A study of adults trying to lose weight found that if they weighed themselves more often, they lost more weight and prevented more weight gain over two years than those who weighed themselves less frequently.

In the first days and weeks, you'll see the numbers drop steadily. After that there are natural plateaus, and that's okay. Consider it a time to consolidate your winnings. Even if the scale doesn't change, you're probably continuing to lose fat and may be gaining muscle as you exercise more. (HoMedics also sells scales that indicate lean body mass, so you can distinguish fat loss from muscle gain.) With the protein in your diet, you should be preserving and even building muscle mass. That prevents you from getting the saggies!

CLOTHING SIZE

Take note of your dress size and pants size. One of the great rewards of the diet is fitting into clothes you haven't worn in years—or buying new clothes to flatter your new physique!

BLOOD PRESSURE

Take your blood pressure. There are inexpensive automatic cuffs available at drugstores if you want to measure your own. Chat with your doctor if you're at all concerned about blood pressure. All the foods on the AD are heart healthy. Chia is especially so: published studies show a blood pressure drop of 6.3 mmHg in patients who added it to their diets. Blood pressure dropped in just about everyone in our trial group. Since blood pressure rises as we get older, this lowering effect should benefit most of you. If you have low blood pressure to begin with, it may get lower, though this hasn't created symptoms for anyone we've tested. I recommend weekly measurements.

BELLY MEASUREMENT

Use a tape measure to determine the circumference of your waist in inches. This is a key measurement for identifying metabolic syndrome, a potentially deadly condition. We want to see belly fat disappear!

Directions

Place a tape measure around your bare abdomen at the level of your hip bones. Don't cheat by holding your breath or sucking in your belly!

Women at risk measure 35 inches or more.
Men at risk measure 40 inches or more.

At those waist measurements, there is not just belly fat, but a full-blown metabolic factory pouring toxic substances throughout the body and the heart's arteries. Take action!

BLOOD WORK

Ask your doctor to order some routine blood work so you'll be able to document your metabolic breakthrough. There's a table of normal values in the Appendix against which to compare. These are the tests I recommend:

- CHOLESTEROL: Complete levels with HDL, LDL, triglycerides. These values should start to fall in response to the Chia Challenge, in as little as five days. Large changes are seen after six weeks.

- FASTING BLOOD SUGAR: This test is the best way to tell if you're prediabetic. If your number is high, expect it to fall quickly. Mine was 99 when I started and is now 83.

- **INFLAMMATION** is responsible for half of all heart disease and a host of other illnesses. People feel terrible in a highly inflammatory state. Ask for a C-reactive protein test, or CRP. This takes a longer, more concerted effort to drop, about two months.

- **A1C:** A long-term marker of blood sugar control, this test is optional unless you have diabetes.

BMI

This is the standard, worldwide measure of obesity and a good indicator of how overweight you are. Use the CDC's BMI calculator at www.cdc.gov.healthyweight/assessing/bmi/adult_bmi/english_bmi_calculator/bmi_calculator.html. All you need is your height and weight.

FOOD LOG

One of the advantages of the AD is that you'll have no need to keep a food log. If you hit a plateau, take a look at your daily carb load. Some of our Chia Challengers, for example, had too much fruit in their smoothies. After they cut it down, their weight continued to drop.

CLEAN THE CUPBOARDS

Time to throw out the junk! Trust me; at 9:00 P.M. I used to scour the cupboards for anything I could devour. Make sure you can't find anything but the premium foods in this book.

REINFORCEMENT

Dieting can be a lonely business, and the biggest reason for dropping out is lack of support. Put together a neighborhood, health club, school group, or work group if you can.

ROAD MAP: SAMPLE DAYS

Below are a couple of sample days to show you what Phase One should look like. If you're a creature of habit, you might be happy having the same smoothie day in and day out. If you need more variety and are home during the day, you can make a different smoothie for every meal since they take only a few minutes to prepare. **All of our recipes make between 2 and 3 cups, which may serve as one meal. The smoothies range in calories, which are listed in the recipes, along with carb load. Women should try to aim for a daily total, including snacks, of about 1,200 calories. Men should aim for a daily total of about 1,600 calories.**

Week 1, Day 1

BREAKFAST: Dr. Bob's Kale Blueberry smoothie (Put your smoothie in a portable water bottle or insulated cup and take it to work with you. Drink it slowly over a couple of hours in the morning.)

LUNCH: Gazpacho Gratitude smoothie

SNACK: ½ cup red quinoa or a few slices low-fat cheese

DINNER: Kale Apple Carrot smoothie

Day 2

BREAKFAST: Strawberries All the Whey smoothie

LUNCH: Pineapple Arugula Macadamia Nut smoothie

SNACK: 1 apple

DINNER: Mango Spinach Ginger smoothie

Up Your Chia

During the first three days, use one scoop of chia in each of your three daily smoothies. (Some brands of chia come with a scooper. One scoop equals 2 tablespoons.) For the rest of the first week, use one and a half scoops (3 tablespoons) of chia in your breakfast smoothie. Stick to one scoop for the lunch and dinner smoothies. In the second week, bump up to two scoops of chia in the morning. Two scoops make a very thick smoothie, so, if you prefer, make your breakfast smoothie with one scoop and mix a second scoop into a glass of water or other low-calorie drink to sip as a morning snack. Throughout Phase One, use only one scoop in your lunch and dinner smoothies. It looks like this:

Chia Chart

DAYS 1–3	DAYS 4–7	WEEK 2
Breakfast smoothie: 1 scoop	Breakfast smoothie: 1½ scoops	Breakfast smoothie: 2 scoops (or 1 scoop in smoothie, 1 scoop in water)
Lunch smoothie: 1 scoop	Lunch smoothie: 1 scoop	Lunch smoothie: 1 scoop
Dinner smoothie: 1 scoop	Dinner smoothie: 1 scoop	Dinner smoothie: 1 scoop

WARNING: If the added fiber and volume of chia cause you to feel bloated or experience heartburn, scale back gradually by quarter scoops until you find the amount that you can tolerate best. Use that amount in your smoothies for three days, then start building back up once your stomach has adjusted. These symptoms are actually a *good* sign and mean that the chia is working to fill you up. If you eat regular foods along with your chia smoothies, you will likely overload your stomach and may experience heartburn. Also, there are those who will not be able to increase their chia. If you have a hiatus hernia or gastric reflux your stomach will become very full. Don't be discouraged; simply reduce the amount of chia you eat.

MAKING SMOOTHIES

Now we'll show you exactly how to make the chia smoothies that will be your breakfast, lunch, and dinner while you're on Phase One, and then you're off and running. There are many different options, but don't get overwhelmed. A host of recipes follow, as well as a detailed guide to concocting your own signature blends. I have my Kale Blueberry chia smoothie every day. It's simple, but it works!

Smoothie Recipes

The first recipe here is for my favorite go-to smoothie, a kale blueberry blend that is filling and chock-full of nutrients. The others hail from culinary duo Mary Corpening Barber and Sara Corpening Whiteford, identical twins who live in California and have made an art of incorporating superfoods into delicious gourmet meals. Some of these recipes originated in their book *Super-Charged Smoothies* but have been altered to meet AD guidelines. Chia smoothies are the ultimate new superfood, offering staggering nutrition in a delicious, super-easy meal.

All of these recipes are best when prepared in a high-speed blender such as a Vitamix. The ultra-powerful engine will blend any fruit or vegetable into a smooth, well-incorporated drink that is more palatable than the chunky results you'll get with a standard blender. (See the FAQs in Chapter 4 for more on high-speed blenders.) The smoothies change drastically over time, so, although you should drink them slowly, they are best served immediately. If you must prepare one in advance to take for lunch, for example, be sure to shake or stir it before drinking. To make your chia more easily digestible, you can let it soak in a glass with ¼ cup of water before adding it to your smoothie.

BREAKFAST

Dr. Bob's Kale Blueberry Smoothie

CALORIES: 334
CARB LOAD: 20

　　1 cup filtered water

　　4 tablespoons chia

　　½ cup plain nonfat Greek yogurt

　　½ cup blueberries

　　3 cups chopped stemmed kale leaves

　　1 teaspoon honey

Combine the water, chia, yogurt, blueberries, kale, and honey in a blender. Blend until smooth.

Melon Mojo

CALORIES: 330
CARB LOAD: 15

　　2 cups diced peeled honeydew melon, chilled

　　1 cup frozen grapes

　　½ cup chopped seeded cucumber, peeled if waxed or bitter

　　¼ cup filtered water

　　2 tablespoons chia

　　1 teaspoon fresh lime juice, plus more as needed

　　12 medium fresh mint leaves

　　Pinch of sea salt

Combine the honeydew, grapes, cucumber, water, chia, lime juice, mint leaves, and sea salt in a blender. Blend until smooth. Add more lime juice if needed.

Strawberries All the Whey

CALORIES: 310
CARB LOAD: 13

   1 cup almond milk

   2 cups fresh or frozen strawberries

   1 scoop (2 tablespoons) whey protein powder

   2 tablespoons chia

   2 teaspoons honey

Combine the almond milk, strawberries, protein powder, chia, and honey in a blender. Blend until smooth.

Note: Also tastes great with peaches!

Blueberry Brain Boost

CALORIES: 472
CARB LOAD: 20.5

   1 cup filtered water

   ½ cup freshly pressed apple juice

   2 tablespoons chia

   ½ ripe banana

   1½ cups fresh or frozen blueberries

   ½ cup fresh or frozen raspberries

   2 tablespoons raw walnuts

Combine the water, apple juice, chia, and banana in a blender. Add the blueberries, raspberries, and walnuts. Blend until smooth.

Note: Cashews are a fine substitute for walnuts if you prefer them.

Jasmine Peach Lassi

CALORIES: 239.5
CARB LOAD: 17.25

    1½ teaspoons raw honey
    ¾ cup warm strong-brewed jasmine tea
    1½ cups diced peaches (skin optional)
    ¾ cup plain low-fat Greek yogurt
    2 tablespoons chia
    4 to 6 ice cubes

Dissolve the honey in the warm tea. Refrigerate until chilled. Combine the sweetened tea, peaches, yogurt, chia, and ice in a blender. Blend until smooth.

Note: This smoothie is best when peaches are at their peak.

Pom Acai

CALORIES: 392.5
CARB LOAD: 22

    ½ cup pomegranate juice
    ½ cup filtered water
    ½ ripe banana
    1 cup fresh or frozen blueberries
    2 tablespoons chia
    One 3½-ounce unsweetened acai smoothie pack (found in supermarkets' frozen fruit section)

Combine the pomegranate juice, water, and banana in the blender. Add the blueberries, chia, and acai smoothie pack. Blend until smooth.

Note: If you can't find the unsweetened acai smoothie pack, add another ½ cup of blueberries or raspberries.

Kale Apple Carrot

CALORIES: 340
CARB LOAD: 20

1½ cups freshly pressed organic carrot juice

½ cup filtered water

1 cup firmly packed chopped stemmed kale leaves

1 small apple, diced (peeled if apple is not organic or skin is waxed)

2 tablespoons raw sunflower seeds

2 tablespoons chia

1 tablespoon fresh lemon juice

Combine the carrot juice, water, kale, apple, sunflower seeds, chia, and lemon juice in a blender. Blend until smooth.

Gazpacho Gratitude

CALORIES: 323.5
CARB LOAD: 14.25

2½ cups cherry tomatoes

2 tablespoons chia

1 medium carrot, peeled and roughly chopped

¾ cup roughly chopped English cucumber

¾ cup roughly chopped peeled cantaloupe

3 tablespoons chopped red onion

1 tablespoon fresh lemon juice

2 teaspoons extra-virgin olive oil

5 medium fresh basil leaves

½ teaspoon sea salt, plus more to taste

Freshly ground pepper

Combine the tomatoes, chia, carrot, cucumber, cantaloupe, red onion, lemon juice, olive oil, basil, sea salt, and pepper to taste in a blender and pulse until smooth but still chunky. Season with more sea salt and pepper to taste.

Apple Cuke Parsley Mint

CALORIES: 317
CARB LOAD: 13.5

    1 cup freshly pressed apple juice

    1 cup filtered water

    2 tablespoons chia

    1 small diced green apple, such as Granny Smith (peeled if apple is not organic or skin is waxed)

    ½ cup roughly chopped cucumber, peeled if waxed or bitter

    1 cup firmly packed fresh parsley leaves

    1 cup firmly packed fresh mint leaves

Combine the apple juice, water, chia, apple, cucumber, parsley, and mint in a blender. Blend until smooth.

Pineapple Arugula Macadamia Nut

CALORIES: 331
CARB LOAD: 13

    1¼ cups filtered water

    ½ cup freshly pressed apple juice

    1½ cups chopped fresh pineapple, chilled

    ¾ cup arugula leaves

    ¾ cup fresh mint leaves

    1 tablespoon roughly chopped raw macadamia nuts

    2 tablespoons chia

    Pinch of sea salt

Combine water, apple juice, pineapple, arugula, mint, macadamia nuts, chia, and salt in a blender. Blend until smooth.

Note: Raw almonds are a fine substitute for macadamia nuts.

Orange Sugar Snap and Pumpkin Seeds

CALORIES: 366
CARB LOAD: 13

> 1 cup orange segments with juice, chilled
>
> 1 cup raw sugar snap peas, tips and strings removed
>
> ½ cup freshly pressed apple juice
>
> 1 cup filtered water
>
> ½ cup fresh mint leaves
>
> 1 tablespoon raw pumpkin seeds
>
> 2 tablespoons chia
>
> 1 teaspoon extra virgin olive oil
>
> Dash of cayenne

Combine the orange segments, sugar snap peas, apple juice, water, mint, pumpkin seeds, chia, olive oil, and cayenne in a blender. Blend until smooth.

Note: This smoothie is at its best in the winter, when citrus is at its peak.

Avo-Colada

CALORIES: 414.5
CARB LOAD: 19

> 1¼ cups coconut water (9.5-fluid-ounce package)
>
> ½ cup chopped ripe avocado
>
> 1¾ cups chopped frozen pineapple
>
> 2 tablespoons chia
>
> 1 tablespoon fresh lime juice
>
> Pinch of sea salt

Combine the coconut water, avocado, pineapple, chia, lime juice, and salt in a blender. Blend until smooth.

Mango Spinach Ginger

CALORIES: 284
CARB LOAD: 13.5

> 1½ cups filtered water
>
> 1½ cups chopped mango
>
> 1 cup spinach
>
> ½ small avocado or ½ cup chopped avocado
>
> 1 teaspoon chopped peeled fresh ginger
>
> 2 tablespoons chia
>
> 1 to 2 teaspoons fresh lemon juice, to taste

Combine the water, mango, spinach, avocado, ginger, chia, and lemon juice. Blend until smooth.

Note: The sweet-tart nature of a mango varies greatly; some are sweet and not tart at all, and some are on the tart side. Add lemon accordingly, and if it is sour add agave nectar or a hint of stevia.

Watermelon Aqua Fresca

CALORIES: 226
CARB LOAD: 13

> 3 cups diced seeded watermelon, chilled
>
> 1 cup spinach
>
> 1 cup frozen strawberries
>
> 2 tablespoons chia
>
> 2 teaspoons fresh lemon juice
>
> 20 fresh mint leaves
>
> Pinch of sea salt

Combine the watermelon, spinach, strawberries, chia, lemon juice, mint, and salt in a blender. Blend until smooth.

Invent Your Own Chia Smoothie

If you're interested in developing your own perfect smoothie, the following guide will explain exactly what you need. Play around with different ingredients to tinker with taste and consistency.

INGREDIENTS

1. The Base

Greek yogurt is our favorite base because it's got a ton of protein, a low carb load, and it adds a silky creaminess to the smoothie with no fat. Fage, Chobani, and Cabot are reliable brands. Use plain yogurt if you're going to add mixers and sweeteners. If you use yogurt with fruit already added, skip the mixer so you don't end up with too much sugar. Most people with lactose intolerance do fine with Greek yogurts, but if they trouble your tummy, try using almond milk.

BASE, 1 CUP	PROTEIN (G)	CALORIES	CL
Greek yogurt (Fage, 0%)	20	120	8
Soy milk	8	131	9
Hemp milk	5	110	5
Almond milk, unsweetened	1	40	0

Research at Appalachian State University shows that whole chia seeds don't work for weight loss. They pass through the digestive system, while the nutrients in ground or sliced chia are readily absorbed. You can put whole seeds in a high-speed blender with your smoothie ingredients, but I buy premium chia microsliced to the precise size that makes it most bioavailable.

2. The Mixer

Mixers aren't necessary if you're using a milk for your base. With a yogurt-based smoothie, however, you'll need a bit of liquid to help your blender churn and make your smoothie drinkable—especially if you're using frozen fruits. A little water always does the trick, but if you're hankering for more flavor or sweetness, try one of the following mixers. Apple juice is the most common mixer in commercial products; it's got a low carb load but not a lot of nutrients. Not to worry, though; those will come with your fruits, veggies, and chia. Grapefruit juice is the lowest-calorie fruit juice. It's high in nutrient density and will help fill you up while keeping your carb load in check.

Our first test group used V8 V-Fusion to add taste and nutrients to their smoothies. If you're worried about your salt intake, buy the low-sodium version or try plain tomato juice. If you want a fizzy, low-cal smoothie, squeeze a quarter of a lime into a cup of sparkling water for your mixer. To keep drudgery at bay it helps to differentiate breakfast smoothies from lunch and dinner smoothies. To that end, some of our innovative dieters have used low-sodium vegetable or chicken broth and even miso soup as mixers.

Ice is always a great addition to a smoothie, and if your blender's up to the task, it can take the place of a mixer. Yogurt, chia, fruit, and ice make for a thick, chilly delight. Whatever you choose, don't feel guilty about adding a sweet mixer to your smoothie to cover up the taste of veggies you would not otherwise eat. Some people carry a special gene that allows them to love the bitter taste of veggies. I'm not one of them. I started out using sweet mixers, but over time my taste weaned away from the supersweet. So will yours as the addiction to sugar is broken.

MIXER, 1 CUP	CALORIES	CL
Water	0	0
Coconut water	46	3
Tomato juice	49	4
Gatorade	50	0
Vegetable juice (V8)	51	4
Carrot juice	94	8
Grapefruit juice (pink)	96	7
Orange juice	112	9
Apple juice	114	6
Pomegranate juice	134	8
Cranberry juice cocktail	137	8

3. Fruits and Veggies

True Aztec fruits include mango, papaya, guava, banana, lime, and orange. Berries bring a lot to the table, as these tiny, tender wonders are packed with flavor as well as antioxidants. Try blueberries, strawberries, raspberries, and blackberries. You don't have to buy fresh; frozen fruits and veggies are often more nutritious, because nutritional value falls steadily on the long journey from farm to grocer. Frozen fruits and veggies are picked at the peak of ripeness, when they're most flavorful, and flash-frozen to lock in nutrients. They make smoothies deliciously cold, thick, and smooth without using ice. I always freeze my kale and other veggies. This makes the smoothie colder and hides the veggie taste.

Bananas impart a fabulous milk shaky texture and therefore are a smoothie staple. Because they carry a higher carb load than other fruits, just use a quarter of a banana. They're sweet enough that a little nugget's all you need. Peel them, cut them up, put them in a plastic zippered bag, and freeze. Turn to our premium foods section (Chapter 8) for tables containing all the numbers you'll need on fruits.

Veggies are great for lunch or dinner smoothies and can disappear into a morning smoothie while fruits take center stage. Hiding veggies is a brilliant way of sneaking crucial nutrients into your diet, and a chia smoothie is the perfect hiding place. Kale is my favorite smoothie veggie. With a perfect ANDI score of 1,000, it is the top-rated vegetable, just brimming with antioxidants. It's got a crisp, tangy flavor that melds nicely with Greek yogurt, providing a sophisticated balance for the sweetness of fruit smoothies. Spinach makes the top five on the ANDI scale, and its velvety texture and mild flavor make it vanish into your smoothie. Were it not for the gorgeous green hue it casts, you'd never know it's there. Broccoli packs a more bitter punch, but it's loaded with soluble fiber, so it's worth working in. You can cloak it in a sweet mixer or try putting it in a gazpacho-like blend for a jolt of nutrition that's delicious and highly enjoyable. Check out the veggie table in Chapter 8 for more of the goods on greens.

4. Chia!

The key with chia is to go ground or microsliced. Whole seeds don't work for weight loss because they sail right through the digestive system and out the other end. Our weight-loss trials reaped great results with microsliced chia because it is maximally bioavailable to the enzymes in the stomach. That means that when the chia hits the stomach, digestive enzymes have maximum access to a greater surface area of chia to better absorb its amazing nutrients and pull them into the bloodstream.

There are many different chia suppliers, so select yours carefully. Seed quality varies enormously from the best high-octane stuff to low-end chia that's thinned with wheat chaff. The best seeds have very high concentrations of omega-3s, protein, and fiber. Bear in mind that dieters have had disappointing results using poor-quality chia or whole seeds, so it's worth finding a reliable source of the good stuff. I've bought whole seeds and ground them, only to feel that my stomach was upset because the quality was poor. See our buyer's guide in the Appendix to get the lay of the land. Look for certified lab results on content.

5. Sweeteners

Again, don't sweat sweetening your smoothie to make it taste better to you. I found that I much prefer using honey and water or ice over fruit juices in my smoothies. Juices tend to add a fake, processed taste that masks the true flavor of fruit. Stevia, a natural, low-CL sweetener made from the leaves of the stevia plant, is a surprisingly effective no-calorie sweetener. Its extracts have 300 times the sweetness of sugar, so a very little bit adds a powerfully sweet punch with no aftertaste. I still like the pure taste of honey best. Only 60 calories per tablespoon, honey accentuates the natural sweetness of fruit without tasting sugary. Give some of the adventurous flavors in the following table a whirl, too. They'll add little to your overall CL but a lot to your pleasure!

FLAVOR	CAL	CARB LOAD
Stevia powder, 1 tablespoon	0	0
Tabasco sauce, 1 teaspoon	1	0
Ginger, fresh, 1 teaspoon	2	0
Cinnamon, 1 tablespoon	19	1
Cocoa powder, unsweetened, 1 tablespoon	20	0
Celery, 2 stalks	36	2
Maple syrup, 1 tablespoon	52	8
Honey, 1 tablespoon	60	10

WHIP IT UP!

Now that you've got your ingredients, you're ready to roll. In a couple of minutes you'll have the healthiest meal on the planet.

Instructions

Put your base and mixer or sweetener, if you're using one, into the blender first. Add chia. Blend the chia, base, and mixer on low speed for a few seconds until incorporated. Stop the blender and add your fruits, veggies, and ice. Blend at high speed until all ingredients are well incorporated. You want your smoothie thick so you can nurse it over a couple of hours, yet thin enough that you can pour it out of the blender.

Ultimately you want a smoothie that you like enough to come back to again and again. If you're concocting your own smoothies, keep these qualities in mind while you're experimenting:

■ MOUTHFEEL is what food companies strive for in designing products. They spend millions getting it just right. Greek yogurt and chia both impart a smooth thickness and terrific mouthfeel. A quarter or half of a banana adds still more. Kale, too, will deliver mouthfeel as well as a jolt of nutrients.

- ■ SWEETNESS: If you're not big on sweets, fruit will be all you need. If you want more, honey, stevia, or fruit juice can turn a veggie blend into a delicious shake. Your total carb load will be so low that you won't be affected by the extra sugar, so make your smoothie taste good!

- ■ THICKNESS: Remember that chia absorbs liquid and expands significantly, so your smoothie will actually get thicker as you sip on it. If you use a milk for your base instead of yogurt, you may want to add thickness with banana or some other fruit. If you want to thin the smoothie, just add ice, water, or other mixer, but beware of slugging down a thin drink too quickly.

> **TIP:** If you're not succeeding in losing weight, cut the amount of juice and/or fruit in your smoothies.

SNACKS

Ideally, you'd eat only chia smoothies during Phase One. Adding snacks does, however, increase compliance, so if you feel you just cannot handle the smoothies without snacking, go right ahead! Choose from our recommended snacks, which we've selected carefully for making you feel full, for low carb load, and for mouthfeel. Don't snack in the morning between your breakfast and lunch smoothies. A 2011 study[1] showed that morning snacking led to more frequent snacking throughout the day and less weight loss than that achieved by those who didn't eat between breakfast and lunch.

Don't snack if you don't need to. You're likely to feel pretty full with the chia smoothies. If you're feeling too full, back off on the amount of chia you add until your body adjusts. If you need to snack, it'll most likely be in the afternoon. Check the snack table for calorie counts and limit the snacks to 200 calories. The table is in ascending order by carb load. Choose snacks with the lowest carb load that will keep you sufficiently full. My favorite afternoon snack is red quinoa! Be wary of the high amounts of omega-6 fats in almonds and pumpkin seeds. Do choose snacks on the higher end of the fullness scale. Forgo evening snacks if you can; we want you to go to bed hungry (in a good way!).

Suggested Snacks

SNACK	OMEGA-6	FULLNESS	CL	ANTI-INFLAMMATION	CALORIES	FIBER	PROTEIN
Almonds, 1 ounce	3,378	2.0	0	51	161	3	6
Celery, 4 medium stalks	87	4.5	0	20	24	4	0
Salsa, 2 tablespoons	0	4.5	0	−4	20	0	0
Pumpkin and squash seeds, 1 ounce	5,326	2.1	0	−24	146	1	9
Beef jerky, 1 ounce	227	2.6	1	5	115	1	9
Light string cheese, 1 piece	100	2.5	1	−13	50	0	6
Hummus, 2 tablespoons	5,005	2.3	2	n/a	50	2	2
Cherry tomatoes, 1 cup	119	4.5	2	14	27	2	1
Carrot sticks, 1 cup	147	3.8	3	199	50	3	1
Edamame, 1 cup	2,781	2.7	6	64	189	8	17
Orange, 1 large	32	3.5	6	9	86	4	2
Nonfat cottage cheese, 1 cup	trace	3.2	6	−30	104	0	15
Apple, 1 large	54	3.3	6	−37	110	3	0
Greek yogurt (Fage 0%), 1 cup	n/a	3.6	8	n/a	120	0	20
Pear, 1 large	43	3.1	8	−47	120	5	1
Rye crackers (Wasa), 1 ounce	>100	2.9	9	−59	94	6	3
Red quinoa, ½ cup	n/a		9		140	5	6
Microwave popcorn, low-fat, 1 ounce	928	2.1	10	−71	119	4	4
Whole wheat crackers (Triscuit), 1 ounce	1,741	1.9	10	−74	124	3	2
All-Bran Multigrain Crackers, 1 ounce	n/a	n/a	est. 10	n/a	120	6	3

Beware: X-Rated Snacks

Here are some conventional snacks that seem pretty healthy, but take a closer look. First, none are very filling, so you're likely to dive back into the bag for more. Second, all of them are inflammatory, especially the granola bar. They all have lots of calories too, for a small serving size. The PowerBar leads the charge at 247 calories. I see overweight gym members ride an exercise bike for 45 minutes, burn 250 calories, then devour a 247-calorie PowerBar. No wonder those guys aren't losing weight! Now look at carb load. PowerBars are through the roof at 29—now THAT is a carb bomb. Great for finishing a mountain climb, but disastrous for dieters. Almost all of these snacks spike your blood sugar with a CL higher than 10. You know there's a lot of fat in the potato chips, but guess what? Trail mix has even more! These are the pitfalls that may have hurt your diet in the past. Now all you have to do is consult the table. Happy snacking!

Snacks to Skip

SNACK	INFLAMMATION	CL	CALORIES	OMEGA-6	FAT
Pretzels, 1 ounce	−107	15	107	322	1
Potato chips, 1 ounce	−73	7	154	3,354	10
Baked potato chips, 1 ounce	−79	12	121	1,130	5
Baked tortilla chips, 1 ounce	−107	15	116	707	2
Trail mix, 1.5 ounces	−71	10	194	4,024	12
PowerBar, 1	−78	29	247	384	2
Fruit leather, 1 ounce	−106	17	104	90	0
Low-fat Granola bar, 1	−145	18	144	1,494	3

THE RECAP

DAYS 1–3:

- Weigh yourself each morning.

- For breakfast, lunch, and dinner, drink a thick smoothie containing *one scoop* of chia.

- Choose an afternoon snack from the suggested list (200 calories or less) and another in the evening if necessary.

DAYS 4–7:

- Weigh yourself each morning.

- For breakfast, drink a thick smoothie containing *one and a half scoops* of chia.

- For lunch and dinner, drink a smoothie containing one scoop of chia.

- Choose an afternoon snack from the suggested list (200 calories or less) and another in the evening if necessary.

WEEK TWO:

- Weigh yourself each morning.

- For breakfast, drink a thick smoothie containing *two scoops* of chia OR a smoothie with one scoop of chia and a second scoop of chia mixed with water or low-calorie beverage.

- For lunch and dinner, drink a smoothie containing one scoop of chia.

- Choose an afternoon snack from the suggested list (200 calories or less) and another in the evening if necessary.

WHEN TO MOVE ON

Move on to Phase Two after two weeks. If you need to lose 20 pounds or more, challenge yourself to stay on Phase One even longer if you can. Moving to Phase Two can boost your metabolism if you reach a plateau, and it will give you more energy for exercise.

CHAPTER 4

LIFE ON PHASE I

AD ALUMNI

By now you have lost a significant amount of weight and should feel utterly fantastic. Your hunger is satisfied, and you're brimming with energy and enthusiasm.

Now that you've stopped spiking your blood sugar with every meal, you've eliminated those devastating crashes. Instead of suffering through several crushing descents each day, you should be feeling smooth, balanced energy. As the numbers on your scale continue to drop, you'll feel lighter and more energetic and, best of all, not starved.

"I felt full all the time, so if I didn't want to eat, I didn't," said Rachel Garcia, a thirty-six-year-old physician's assistant from Jacksonville, Florida. "It felt like my stomach had shrunk. I didn't eat large portions anymore. I just ate what I should eat." Introduced to chia by her brother in 2008, Rachel started eating it for its high omega-3 count. She put a scoop into her breakfast smoothie every morning, and after three months she'd lost 30 pounds, dropping from a size 14 to a size 8.

In 2010, Rachel and her friend Gail Dawson, a mediation attorney, went to a chia event in West Palm Beach, where Rachel and I were speakers. I told the story of my own weight loss after eating four scoops of chia a day. "I can do anything for thirty days," Gail told Rachel on the way home. She had concocted her own chia smoothie of frozen fruit, juice, whey protein, and chia and drank it three times a day in place of meals. In twenty-six days, Gail, fifty-five, lost 24 pounds.

This is how the first Chia Challenge began. Gail shared the plan with Lucy Ann Hoover, a retired FBI agent recently returned from work in Afghanistan, and Lucy experienced the same incredible success, losing 30 pounds and dropping from a size 14 to a size 6. As these women shared their experience, something of a sensation began. Rachel, who works with a plastic surgeon, sees hundreds of clients a week, most of whom would love to return to a single-digit dress size. She soon had dozens of people losing weight with chia smoothies. Together we launched a study to track their progress with the help of Dr. Ellan Duke, a local chiropractor who lent us the use of her office space for blood work and weigh-ins.

The results surpassed everyone's wildest expectations. Participants who stuck with the plan, in essence Phase One of the Aztec Diet, and exercised lost 1 pound a day. Those who didn't exercise lost, on average, ½ pound per day. Not only did these people shed weight at will, their health blossomed. Their blood pressure dropped, their cholesterol dropped, their blood sugar came into the normal range. Fat came off like it had been stripped off with a knife.

As the dieters celebrated their weight loss, a bigger picture began to emerge of a novel and highly effective solution to the obesity epidemic that plagues America: chia. Three weight-loss drugs had recently been banned by the FDA. Here was something far better than any drug: a healthy, raw whole food that controls appetite and aids in weight loss.

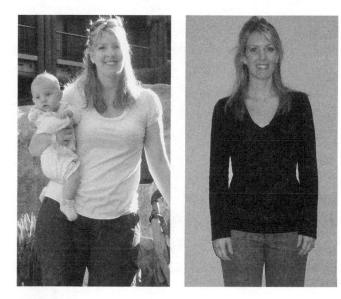

Rachel Garcia

36, Jacksonville, FL

Beginning weight: 165 pounds

End weight: 135 pounds

Weight lost: 30 pounds

Size 14 to size 8

"I felt full all the time, so if I didn't want to eat, I didn't."

Gail Dawson

55, Jacksonville, FL

Beginning weight: 168 pounds

End weight: 144 pounds

Weight lost: 24 pounds

Three chia smoothies a day helped Gail's neck and shoulder pain vanish. Her clinical depression lifted. Hot flashes ceased. She stopped taking ibuprofen, fish oil, and flax. She has also used chia to rehabilitate sick and malnourished dogs.

"I lost 24 pounds in 26 days. I'm thrilled with how I feel."

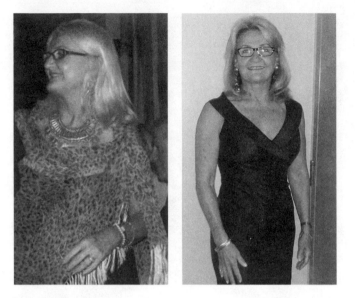

Lucy Ann Hoover
59, Jacksonville, FL
Beginning weight: 175
End weight: 145
Weight lost: 30 pounds
Size 14 to size 6

"I feel more alert and less tired, mentally and physically. I have increased stamina which results in more satisfying workouts."

Oreann White
54, Warwick, Bermuda
Beginning weight: 242 pounds
End weight: 197 pounds
Weight lost: 45 pounds

"My pain has gone away. My cravings have gone away. My mood is better!"

One of the greatest benefits of losing weight on the Aztec Diet is a noticeable increase in energy. Oreann White, a fifty-four-year-old accountant in Bermuda, said she felt the difference within days. After just three days of eating chia, said Oreann, "I noticed the energy. I was running up the steps. I was more alert."

When a customer at the car dealership where Oreann works told her about chia, she had just been to the doctor, who'd told her she was borderline diabetic and must either lose weight or add more medication to the bevy of pills she already took for high blood pressure and cholesterol. No more, said Oreann, who then weighed 242 pounds. She began eating chia right away, on a regimen similar to Phase Two of the AD. After three months of drinking two chia smoothies a day she'd lost 35 pounds. Working somewhat in reverse, she began Phase One of the AD (three smoothies a day) in February 2012 and, after two weeks, had lost 10 more pounds.

Now, Oreann added, "My pain has gone away. My cravings have gone away. My mood is better," she said. "Sometimes God sends stuff along and you have to pay attention!"

Give yourself some well-deserved congratulations. Breaking your old eating habits has probably been tough. Foods are the most popular addictions of our time. They trigger the same responses in the brain as sex, gambling, and recreational drugs, providing a steady series of highs throughout the day. This druglike effect is the biggest reason we overeat, and it's a powerful force to overcome. You've done it!

FREQUENTLY ASKED QUESTIONS

My smoothies aren't smooth; they're chunky! What should I do?

If you can, invest in a high-speed blender such as a Vitamix. They're very pricey, at nearly $400 for the basic model, but will grind nearly any fruit or vegetable into a smooth, palatable blend. These blenders will allow you great variation in your smoothies and are also good for making soups and salad dressings. With a motor like a small lawnmower, this thing will last for years, even when used three times a day.

If the high-speed blender isn't an option, try using fresh fruit instead of frozen. Dice vegetables into smaller pieces and soak nuts in water before adding to your blender. Blend longer, stopping to stir occasionally.

My weight loss slowed down after a couple of weeks. How do I keep losing?

Cut down on the amount of sugar in your smoothies. The carb load may be too high to allow for weight loss if there is too much fruit or fruit juice in your smoothies. Try using water instead of juice and add a squirt of honey or a pinch of stevia if you need a sweetener. Add as many vegetables as you like. Also, this is a great time to add exercise to your routine since you'll now have the energy you need.

I feel bloated and burpy after drinking my chia smoothie. What should I do?

Chia has tons of great fiber and expands in your stomach as it absorbs liquid, so it may take you a little while to adjust to it. Reduce the amount of chia in your smoothies by a quarter of a scoop until you find the amount you can eat comfortably. Stick with that amount for three days, then increase by a quarter scoop at similar intervals until you've reached at least a whole scoop. For those with small stomachs and not much weight to lose, one scoop per smoothie may be enough throughout Phase One. Should you have gastric reflux and suffer heartburn, again, back off on the amount of chia you're adding and drink smaller portions. Chia does fill you up, and can "overfill" you, so customize your approach based on how you feel. Chia is also a tremendous aid to intestinal transport. Many who eat it rave about improved bowel movement.

Do I need to worry about bleeding with chia?

No, chia affects bleeding time in a favorable way in terms of heart attack prevention. However, if you are going to have surgery or are taking a blood-thinning medication, be sure to tell your doctor that you are eating chia.

BENEFITS OF THE AZTEC DIET

Any time you need a little encouragement to stick with the program, flip through these pages to remind yourself of the incredibly good things you're doing for yourself. The benefits you're reaping from the Aztec Diet go far beyond weight loss. You may have noticed some of them already; if not, you soon will.

Find Calm Energy

As you've seen, the biggest single difference you feel on the AD is energy. Lots of it, more than you've ever had, more than you've ever imagined. While most dieters slowly grind to a crawl on bleak, calorie-deprived diets, you're ready to take on more than you ever have. Smoothing out your blood sugar levels and eating a staggering amount of super-nutrients allows your energy stores to skyrocket, a phenomenon proven by the long-distance running prowess of the Tarahumara Indians, for whom chia was a staple food.

Make Your Brain Feel Great

We looked in depth at this in Chapter 2, learning how healthy foods with high amounts of omega-3s enhance the all-important coating of your neurons for superior nerve conduction and neurotransmitter production. Increasing your intake of omega-3s will make you feel noticeably smarter. Chia has more omega-3s than any food on the planet.

Have Better Sex

As you lose weight your sex life will soar. Your self-image will improve, your libido will increase, and even your performance will get a boost. A modest loss of weight, just 5 percent, leads to improvement in erectile dysfunction and increases desire, Australian researchers report. In men with high blood sugar and cholesterol levels and the beginning of diabetes, the small blood vessels in the penis begin to narrow, choking the supply of blood, thus preventing a strong erection. Women suffer too as blood flow slows to a trickle in the small vessels of the clitoris. Susan Kellogg, PhD, director of sexual medicine at the Pelvic and Sexual Health Institute of Graduate Hospital in Philadelphia, has said that this diminished blood flow decreases sexual responsiveness in women.

For men and women, being overweight makes sex hormones less available because they become tied up with binding globulins. Weight loss releases these vital sex hormones, so desire and performance are magnified.

Improve Your Blood Sugar Levels

As we've said, high carb load is the largest health epidemic in America. Most Americans whose high carb load has progressed to prediabetes are blind to the condition. They have no idea they're sick even as they edge toward full-blown diabetes. Even young, healthy athletes struggle to manage carb load. Rare is the person who isn't struggling with it, and that person is probably on the AD!

Whether you have diabetes, prediabetes, or are a healthy, fit person who just can't handle the high carb load of your diet, the AD will help you improve your blood sugar levels. This is the fundamental reward of the AD.

We ran blood work on our first group of dieters and found substantial decreases in:

- fasting blood sugar

- A1C (A long-term measure of blood sugar control, A1C is an important marker. While you may not have outrageously high blood sugar levels at a given time, A1C keeps score of your overall average.)

- waist circumference (a good measure of decreased belly fat)

- blood pressure (a key part of a lethal blood sugar problem called *metabolic syndrome*)

Staggering though it may seem, more Americans have problems with their blood sugar levels than are obese. There are 72 million obese Americans but 82.2 million with blood sugar problems. Here are more sobering numbers:

- Americans with prediabetes: 57 million

- Americans with diabetes: 25.8 million

Of those cases, only an estimated 18.8 million are diagnosed, leaving 7 million undiagnosed.

Though we're wary of making outrageous claims, it does appear that most traces of adult-onset diabetes vanish on the Aztec Diet. The Harvard School of Public Health estimates that 85 percent of type II diabetes can be prevented, and I totally agree. In fact, I strongly object to the medicalization of what is really a lifestyle disease. I have talked with diabetics who are consumed with doctor visits, blood tests, and prescription drugs but totally ignore the fact that they suffer from a lifestyle disease and are doing little to remedy it. We have found astonishing results with diabetics reducing or stopping their insulin entirely, under their doctor's direction.

Hopefully you had your blood sugar levels measured before beginning the diet; now you can watch them decline steadily. My own blood sugar dropped from 99, nearly prediabetic, to 82 on the AD. (A person with a fasting blood sugar level of 100 is considered prediabetic; 125 indicates diabetes.)

Boost Your Metabolism

Many studies show that, even with exercise, diets cause patients' metabolic rates to fall. The reason for this slowing metabolism is that the diets don't supply enough calories at the right times of day. The AD strategically inputs calories in the four-hour window before exercise or other major activity to boost your metabolism and take off pounds. The AD manages your metabolism so that you can have calm energy in the morning and evening and incredible physical energy for your workout.

Improve Your Mood

Famed MIT researcher Judith Wurtman, author of *Managing Your Mind and Mood Through Food*, pioneered the idea that the foods we eat influence the kinds of neurochemicals our brains produce. For instance, pure protein promotes the production of highly energizing adrenalinelike neurochemicals, whereas carbohydrates produce calming ones like serotonin. Using the right foods at the right time of day is critical to managing your mood. Eating protein in the morning energizes your brain; eating carbohydrates in the midafternoon allows you to settle down when your brain is most likely to.

We've engineered the AD to provide you with the right neurotransmitters at the right time of day. The diet also boosts your mood by keeping your blood sugar level and supplying your brain with a steady energy supply. Foods that encourage a good night's sleep also play a huge role in brightening your day.

Banish Belly Fat

The AD first and foremost targets belly fat. This is the fat that kills you. My 18-year-old son, Hayden, is an amazing oarsman and very fit. He constantly asks me, however, "Dad, how do I get rid of belly fat?" I tell him that he suffers from carb overload, which opens up the cells around his belly and pours in the fat. Carb overload increases the risk of central obesity and the development of the deadly metabolic syndrome. The solution: back off of the wrong carbs, eat the right fat, and the belly fat will vanish. Belly fat is also the key marker of inflammation throughout your body. As you drive inflammation down by eating anti-inflammatory foods, your belly fat will disappear. Some of the foods on the AD are especially good belly fat busters, such as Greek yogurt. Belly-fat-burning exercises help too. Believe me, washboard abs are not an impossibility!

Heal Your Heart

We ran tests for heart health on our first group of AD dieters. Here are the amazing findings:

LOWERED BLOOD PRESSURE

Blood pressure fell in everyone. Since nearly all of us will become hypertensive with age, this is a great benefit of the AD. Although BP has taken a backseat to cholesterol in the public's mind, it's an incredibly important risk factor for stroke as well as heart disease. BP is much more pleasantly controlled with diet than with drugs. Frank Sacks, MD, a cardiologist at the Harvard School of Public Health, says, "Diets lower blood pressure more than most drugs." Blood pressure is expressed as two numbers (e.g., 120/80). The systolic number is the first one and the most important. Published data[1] on one strain of chia showed a 6.3 mmHg drop in systolic blood pressure in those who ate it. A systolic drop of 6 mmHg is quite significant. To go from 130 to 124, for example, would make your doctor very happy! Part of the plunge is thanks to the enormous drop in salt consumption on the AD; the addition of blood-pressure-friendly minerals such as potassium, calcium, and magnesium helps too.

LOWERED LDL ("BAD") CHOLESTEROL

This is one of the early and most significant metabolic changes brought on by the AD. After two weeks you should see a pretty significant drop in LDL. My friend Dean Ornish says, if you haven't succeeded in lowering your cholesterol with diet, then double down! In other words, make much more intensive dietary efforts. Chances are that you'll succeed. Many of Dean's patients have done as well with diet as they have with medication. New studies back him up with positive results rivaling those achieved with medications.

A NOTE ABOUT MEDICATIONS: We found that some dieters dropped their LDL enough that they considered stopping their cholesterol medications. I don't recommend this unless your doctor concurs, since there are other key protective qualities of these medications, such as plaque stabilization. Most heart attacks are not caused by a clogged artery; they're caused by a piece of plaque that breaks off from the artery wall. This results in the complete occlusion of the artery and the death of heart muscle. Statins continue to protect you against this catastrophic event by preventing the caps on these plaques from loosening and pouring highly inflammatory cholesterol into your arteries. The anti-inflammatory foods of the AD may lower your body's inflammation level enough to reconsider your meds, but only with your doctor's approval.

LOWERED DAMAGING TRIGLYCERIDES

Though not as well known a villain as cholesterol, triglycerides are an incredibly important blood fat. Carb overload will make your TRG levels soar. Our dieters found that TRG levels plummeted within the first two weeks on the AD.

FEWER IRREGULAR HEARTBEATS

Many of us notice a skipped or irregular beat at quiet times, and it worries us. A key benefit of the omega-3 fatty acids in the AD is that they can decrease irregular heartbeats called *arrhythmias*. I notice no skipped beats when I stick strictly to the AD. A Harvard School of Public Health study showed decreased risk of atrial fibrillation with a high omega-3 intake.[2]

LOWERED INFLAMMATION

At least half of heart disease is due to inflammation. We measured CRP (C-reactive protein), a key indicator of inflammation. Within six weeks this hard-to-move marker had begun to fall. When you eat the anti-inflammatory foods of the AD, you'll find that the fire within ceases to smolder. This is a great measure of your success.

DECREASED HEART FAILURE

A new Harvard study[3] shows that for people with good levels of omega-3 fatty acids the incidence of heart failure is cut in half. The AD is rich in omega-3s.[4]

Live Longer!

Okay, this may be the most fascinating of all. A little thing called the *telomere* protects the ends of chromosomes from the deterioration that occurs with aging. The telomere shortens with each cell replication. So, over time, the shorter the telomere, the more likely we are to succumb to disease and eventually die. It's like an aging fuse. When the last of the fuse vanishes, the organism dies. A study of women published in the *American Journal of Clinical Nutrition* showed that those with better body composition (e.g., less fat) and a great diet, including cereal fiber, had the longest telomere lengths.[5] The higher the linoleic acid and waist circumference, the shorter the telomere length. Fascinating!

Walk, Don't Waddle

There's a distinctive waddle that plagues the obese. Walk into any amusement park in America and you'll see scores of the obese who waddle. Nobody talks about this. Nobody talks about chafing legs or the maddening inability to do anything or get anywhere fast. It's uncomfortable, unsightly, and embarrassing. It seems simple but worth pointing out: lose weight, lose the waddle. After a weight loss of 27 percent, subjects in a study published in the *Journal of Applied Physiology* walked 3.9 percent faster.[6] After an additional 6.5 percent weight loss they became 7.3 percent faster. All aspects of gait improved, including stride length, hip range of motion, maximal knee flexion, and ankle flexion. That alone is worth getting going. Walk on!

Improve Cell Function

We really are what we eat, right down to the cellular level. Each cell has a wall made largely from fats. The kind of fats you eat determines the kind of fats contained in that wall. When you eat large amounts of omega-6 fatty acids, these are incorporated into the cell wall and the chemicals inside become a toxic stew of inflammatory substances. Membranes made of omega-3 fatty acids function far better. The chemicals inside are no longer angry, and the cell stops making inflammatory products.

- One example of this lies in the pain pathway. Your body feels more pain when you have large amounts of omega-6 fatty acids and less when you have large amounts of omega-3s. The cascade of omega-6s sneaking in with your salad dressing summons a long list of bad actors that increase pain. Cut omega-6s and up the omega-3s to shut down the production of these pain products.

- Another example lies in the breast duct cell where breast cancers form. When cells contain high levels of omega-6s, they become hyperresponsive to estrogen. The more responsive the cells are to estrogen, the more fuel is added to the growth of existing breast cancer cells. High levels of omega-3s, on the other hand, dampen the cells' response to estrogen. Dr. John Glaspy concluded that omega-6 fatty acids "may be contributing to the high risk of breast cancer in the United States and that LC n-3 PUFAs, derived from fish oils, may have a protective effect."

Feel Young, Look Young, Act Young!

I've been on the Aztec Diet for nearly two years. The most remarkable thing about the diet for me is how young I feel, look, and act. I've long believed that most signs of aging actually come from abuse, and now I'm sure of it. I compete in ski races, long-distance bike races, and surfing competitions with kids who are 40 years younger, and I sometimes win! I recently crossed the 32-mile channel between Molokai and Oahu on a paddleboard using chia as my primary fuel. I've just never felt better. Pouring inflammatory foods and carb bombs into our bodies speeds up the aging process. High blood sugar levels fray the basic building blocks of the body's collagen fibers. Inflammation physically destroys tissues, from the brain and lungs to the arteries in the heart. Many Americans look, act, and feel far older than they are. Don't let that be you. Stay on the AD and defy aging.

MOVING ON

The next chapter will show you how to move on to Phase Two. If you really can't hang on to Phase One for two weeks, don't quit! Begin Phase Two rather than return to your old eating patterns.

If you opt to stay on Phase One for longer than two weeks, there are a few developments that will signal when you're ready to move on:

1. You hit a plateau and your weight loss slows considerably. Phase Two replaces the lunch smoothie with a high-protein meal that will give your metabolism a well-timed boost.

2. You've lost as much weight as you want. Even if you're where you want to be, use Phase Two as a gradual return to solid food. This phase ensures that you eat the bulk of your calories at the right times of day so you don't regain weight.

3. You want to exercise and need more energy. Eating a meal of vegetables, low-CL grains, and lean protein at midday will fuel an intense late-afternoon workout. By the time you leave work your food will be digested and you won't sabotage your sleep or your waistline with a big meal before you sleep.

PHASE II

PHASE TWO OF THE AZTEC DIET: SIX WEEKS

- The Plan: A Chia Smoothie for Breakfast; Lunch of Veggies, Low-CL Grains, and Lean Protein; a Chia Smoothie for Dinner

  - Road Map: A Sample Day

    - Lunchtime!

  - When to Move On

LIFE ON PHASE TWO

  - AD Alumni

  - Exercise

- Frequently Asked Questions

  - Moving On

CHAPTER 5

PHASE II: ACCELERATE WITH LUNCH

THE PLAN: A CHIA SMOOTHIE FOR BREAKFAST; SOLID LUNCH; CHIA SMOOTHIE FOR DINNER

Many weight-loss programs give you a good first two weeks or so. The weight peels off, but then you hit a wall. The scales don't budge. You're stuck on the classic dieter's plateau because your metabolism has slowed. This is where Phase Two of the AD changes the game. In Phase Two you continue with chia smoothies for breakfast and dinner but replace the lunchtime smoothie with a high-energy meal. This well-timed influx of calories brings your metabolism roaring back and delivers a jolt of energy for your afternoon workouts.

Phase Two is vitally important, so don't skip it. When you stop drinking smoothies and eat your first real meal, your metabolism roars back. If your old eating pattern also roars back, with it will come a rapid weight gain, and all your effort will be erased. This is why it is important to follow our Phase Two plan.

Don't be tempted to replace the dinner smoothie with a meal instead of lunch either. Phase Two of the AD mimics the eating schedule of the Aztecs, whose main meal was at midday, for good reason. Whether dieting or not, your digestive system shouldn't be saddled with its largest load of food at night, which disturbs sleep patterns and packs on the pounds. Eating at lunchtime allows time for food to digest before an afternoon workout (see Chapter 6) so your exercise burns more fat and leaves you relaxed for the evening. By returning to a smoothie at night, you curb the tendency to start overeating.

I recommend staying on Phase Two for six weeks. This will help you establish new, healthy eating habits and break the old cycle of ending the day with a big dinner.

PHASE TWO

SIX WEEKS

BREAKFAST: Smoothie with 2 scoops of chia, or smoothie with 1 scoop plus water with 1 scoop

LUNCH: Lean protein, low-CL grains and veggies, about 400 calories

DINNER: Smoothie with 1 scoop of chia

In researching what you should eat for that all-important lunch, we found inspiration in the diets of the world's most successful cultures. A few civilizations throughout history grew vast empires based on strength, energy, determination, and a fabulous diet. These diets not only kept populations lean and fit; they also held at bay chronic illnesses such as heart disease, diabetes, and cancer. The Mediterranean diet, considered one of the world's healthiest, gave rise to the ancient Greek civilization and the Roman Empire. The Asian food pyramid spawned the enormous successes of the Japanese and Chinese cultures over the centuries.

These successes weren't coincidental; civilizations flourished in large part because their people ate amazing foods. Oldways Preservation and Trust, a well-known food think tank, in partnership with the Harvard School of Public Health, chronicled, studied, and promulgated these important diets. Oldways created the Mediterranean Pyramid and helped establish it as the most widely recommended diet worldwide.

Dunn Gifford, founder of Oldways, was the ultimate judge of diets and a great inspiration for many of the books and news reports I've written. Gifford helped create the Latin American Pyramid, which ranks alongside the Mediterranean and Asian diets as one of the world's healthiest. At its core lies the original Aztec diet. Stripped of the Columbian and South American influences, Dunn said, "A pure Aztec diet could be the greatest diet of all."

The Aztec diet and others like it included far less variety than we have today. Our abundant choices of processed, high-sugar foods have led us astray. In an age of tremendous food misrepresentation and even outright fraud in advertising and marketing, it's tough to know exactly what you're eating and the damage it can do. Even FDA labels can be hugely misleading. With no way of knowing how much extra sugar, fat, and salt have been packed into the restaurant dishes you eat or the packaged foods you buy, you can unknowingly eat hundreds of extra calories a day.

With Phase Two of the AD, we are going to cut down on variety to make things simpler. With simple choices you'll find it infinitely easier to lose weight. Most diet books are crammed with nearly encyclopedic lists of food choices. You won't find those here. The AD recommends only premium foods with incredible nutritional values. We've carefully researched foods, meticulously checking them across many databases before recommending them for the AD.

Chapter 9 contains many more meals and recipes, but in this chapter you'll find a quick list of lunches that include fish, chicken or turkey, vegetables, and low-CL grains. These foods allow us to add two important ingredients to your diet. First are the omega-3 fatty acids that are so beneficial to your mood and mental well-being. We'll add these with several servings of fish a week, preferably wild Pacific salmon. Next come incredibly powerful antioxidants.

In Phase One you dumped the outrageously inflammatory foods that are responsible for catastrophic illnesses from heart disease to cancer. In Phase Two you'll add foods that will raise your anti-inflammatory level to further protect you from those ailments.

To be clear, we're not talking about a heavy lunch, but one that pumps up your metabolism and energy level without the deadening effects of a high carbohydrate load. Aim to eat about 400 calories at lunch. Men may eat a bit more, women a bit less. The meal suggestions that follow are all within range.

ROAD MAP

Sample Day

BREAKFAST: **Dr. Bob's Kale Blueberry smoothie with 2 scoops of chia**

LUNCH: **Fish tacos**

SNACK: **Carrot sticks and hummus**

DINNER: **Apple Cuke Parsley Mint smoothie with 1 scoop of chia**

LUNCHTIME!

We highly recommend that you select some of the fantastic lunches in Phase Two. If you're pinched for time, however, the following are quick and simple lunch options. The numbers listed after the ingredients refer to CL and calories, respectively.

Spinach Salad

CALORIES: 353
CARB LOAD: 15.5

2 cups spinach (0, 14)

1 cup sliced strawberries (3, 53)

2 tablespoons sliced almonds (0, 104)

½ cup Great Northern or other white beans (7.5, 104)

¼ cup chopped red onion (1, 16)

2 tablespoons low-fat honey mustard dressing, like Annie's Lite Honey Mustard (4, 62) or, better yet, make your own from the dressing recipes in Chapter 9.

Variations

Add 3 ounces cooked chicken (0, 136)

Add 3 ounces cooked shrimp (0, 84)

Add 3 ounces cooked salmon (0, 196)

Add ½ cup quinoa (9, 111)

Egg Salad Sandwich

CALORIES: 384
CARB LOAD: 14

2 hard-boiled eggs (0, 140)

¼ to ½ cup Greek yogurt (4, 60)

¼ cup chopped celery (0, 4)

2 slices sprouted wheat bread, Alvarado Street Bakery (10, 180)

Bean Burger

CALORIES: 260
CARB LOAD: 14

1 black bean or veggie burger (4, 120)

1 Flatout or similar brand low-calorie flatbread, pita, or tortilla (est. 6, 90)

¼ cup or 2 leaves green lettuce (0, 5)

1 slice onion (0, 5)

1 slice tomato (0, 10)

2 tablespoons ketchup (4, 30)

Tuna Salad Sandwich

CALORIES: 380
CARB LOAD: 14

3 ounces canned light tuna (0, 100)

¼ to ½ cup Greek yogurt (4, 60)

¼ cup chopped celery (0, 40)

2 slices sprouted wheat bread, Alvarado Street Bakery (10, 180)

Hummus in a Pita with Lettuce, Tomato, and Red Onion

CALORIES: 221

CARB LOAD: 11

- ¼ cup hummus (4, 100)
- 1 Flatout or similar brand low-calorie flatbread, pita, or tortilla (est. 6, 90)
- ¼ cup lettuce (0, 5)
- 2 slices tomato (0, 10)
- ¼ cup chopped red onion (1, 16)

Chicken Stir-Fry with Brown Rice

CALORIES: 416

CARB LOAD: 15

- 3 ounces cooked chicken (0, 136)
- 1 cup frozen broccoli, thawed (4, 52)
- 1 tablespoon olive oil (0, 120)
- ½ cup cooked brown rice (11, 108)

Variations

Substitute salmon for chicken: Add 60 calories

Substitute turkey for chicken: Subtract 16 calories

Fish Tacos

CALORIES: 268

CARB LOAD: 12

- 2 small corn tortillas (10, 104)
- 3 ounces steamed halibut (0, 120)
- ½ cup shredded green cabbage (1, 8)
- ¼ cup chopped red onion (1, 16)
- 2 tablespoons salsa (0, 20)

Bean Burrito

CALORIES: 340
CARB LOAD: 15

½ cup cooked black beans (7, 114)

1 Flatout or similar brand low-calorie flatbread, pita, or tortilla (est. 6, 90)

¼ cup grated part-skim mozzarella (1, 85)

¼ cup chopped lettuce (0, 5)

2 slices tomato (0, 10)

¼ cup chopped red onion (1, 16)

2 tablespoons salsa (0, 20)

Turkey Sandwich

CALORIES: 326
CARB LOAD: 10

3 ounces roasted turkey, not deli (0, 120)

2 leaves green lettuce (0, 5)

2 slices onion (0, 5)

2 slices tomato (0, 10)

2 slices sprouted wheat bread, Alvarado Street Bakery (10, 180)

2 teaspoons mustard (0, 6)

Turkey-Bean Wrap

CALORIES: 355
CARB LOAD: 14

3 ounces roasted turkey, not deli (0, 120)

½ cup black beans (7, 114)

1 Flatout or similar brand low-calorie flatbread, pita, or tortilla (est. 6, 90)

¼ cup chopped lettuce (0, 5)

2 slices tomato (0, 10)

¼ cup chopped red onion (1, 16)

THE RECAP

PHASE TWO (SIX WEEKS):

- Continue to weigh yourself each morning.

- For breakfast, drink a thick smoothie containing *two scoops* of chia or a smoothie with one scoop and a second scoop in water.

- For lunch, eat a healthy, high-protein lunch of about 400 calories.

- Incorporate exercise in the late afternoon as many days as possible.

- Choose an afternoon snack from the suggested list on page 48 (200 calories or less) and another in the evening if necessary.

- For dinner, drink a smoothie containing one scoop of chia.

WHEN TO MOVE ON

After six weeks on Phase Two, move on to Phase Three, which will return you to three meals a day.

CHAPTER 6

LIFE ON PHASE II

AD ALUMNI

Ridding your body of inflammatory, fattening foods in Phase One probably helped you feel better than you have in years. In Phase Two you'll feel even better, enjoying the satisfaction of a solid midday meal and the many benefits of blood-pumping exercise. Your chia smoothie continues to carry you through the morning on a tide of amazing nutrients, so you won't be driven by hunger to make unwise choices for your lunch.

"I've never been able to do any kind of diet consistently," said Jack Galante, owner of a construction company in San Jose, California. But because he didn't feel hungry,

Jack was able to stick with the Aztec Diet. As weight fell away, he was most amazed by the fact that his cravings for beer, burgers, and ice cream were gone. "It's not difficult," he said. "I have no desire for them!"

Jack got his wake-up call when, facing his fourth knee replacement and suffering from high cholesterol, an old friend saw a photo of him on Facebook. "Your face really blew up," wrote the friend. "What are you doing?" Never overweight before, Jack had let the pounds stack up over the last few years. The fifty-six-year-old's diet resembled that of many Americans: coffee and a couple of doughnuts for breakfast; a cheeseburger, fries, soda, and cookies for lunch; a little candy in the afternoon; a couple of beers after work; steak or spaghetti and several pieces of bread for dinner; and a bowl or two of ice cream in the evening.

"I went home and looked in the mirror and thought, 'You better do something,' " Jack said. And he did. After eight weeks on the Aztec Diet, Jack had lost 33 pounds. Starting out at 224 pounds, his goal had been to get under 200 pounds. Having reached 191, he visited his doctor. His medical file showed that just three years earlier he'd weighed 187 pounds. "I can get back there!" he said enthusiastically, "No problem!" By then Jack's wife had lost 23 pounds and five of his friends had started the diet. "I haven't had beer in three months," Jack said. "I have no desire. I get out of bed and have more energy than I've had in I can't tell you how long."

Jack Galante
56, San Jose, CA
Beginning weight: 224 pounds
End weight: 191 pounds
Weight lost: 33 pounds

"Getting on the scale every day works. It tells you what you've done wrong the day before. I wanted to lose weight and feel better, and it's not difficult. It works."

Sonya Campos
42, Santa Clara, CA
Beginning weight: 325
Still going!
Weight lost: 30 pounds

"Pain doesn't hold me back."

Sonya Campos, a forty-two-year-old manager of a credit union in Santa Clara, California, kicked a habit of drinking four large cans of Red Bull a day when the chia smoothie helped kill her cravings for caffeine and sugar. Starting out at 325 pounds, Sonya has already lost 30 pounds and hopes to lose 100 more. "Life has led me astray, and I'm trying to get back," said Sonya.

Beset with pain before she encountered chia, Sonya said everything in her body hurt. Doctors had recommended hormone therapy, pain medications, and chiropractic realignment. Instead, Sonya started drinking chia smoothies in June 2011. She had blood work done in August, and her doctor found that her cholesterol and blood sugar were well controlled and other labs had normalized. "When I don't eat my chia, I'm in pain," Sonya said. "When I do eat it, pain doesn't hold me back. I'm living life and not complaining constantly that I don't feel good."

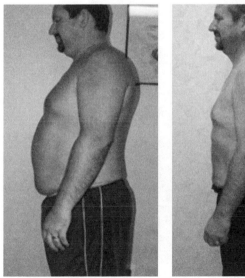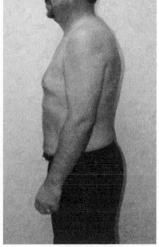

Ian Fraser
43, Jacksonville, FL
Beginning weight: 244 pounds
End weight: 203 pounds
Weight lost: 41 pounds
Cholesterol: 174 to 162
Blood pressure: 118/90 to 102/70

Now that you're well on your way to your target weight, it's possible to see how the pounds you've shed were affecting your life. Without them your body is lighter, more agile, and more energetic. But you may be relieved by the lifting of a psychological burden as well.

At an event held at the end of the first Chia Challenge in Orlando, Florida, in 2010, the projector showed photographs of one of the winners, Ian Fraser, at his heaviest: 244 pounds. When Ian walked onstage, he looked transformed at 203 pounds. Ian helped me understand the degree to which overweight people are ostracized. Deeply moved, he told the audience how much his life had changed. People didn't sneer at him anymore. They didn't steer a wide course around him. People treated him better. They showed him respect. They didn't ignore him. They wanted to befriend him. Ian had a whole new take on life!

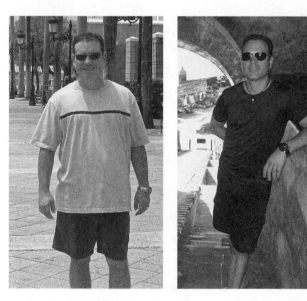

Dr. Francisco Gutierrez
46, Middletown, RI
Beginning weight: 185 pounds
End weight 142 pounds
Weight lost: 43 pounds
Cholesterol: 300 to 202

Dr. Gutierrez's wife, Eleonora, also lost weight on the plan. She is now 20 pounds lighter!

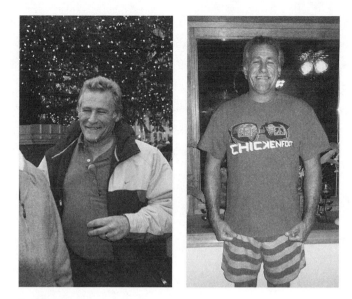

Paul Henriques
49, Portsmouth, RI
Beginning weight: 188 pounds
End weight 168 pounds
Weight lost: 20 pounds

A diabetic, Paul required more than 100 units of insulin via pump each day with consistent monitoring until January 2012. He now requires only 10 units of insulin a day via one injection. His pump was discontinued.

As Jack Galante quickly realized, life on Phase Two feels so good that returning to old eating habits truly loses its appeal. I like to stay on a modified Phase Two pretty much all year. I have a chia smoothie for breakfast, a solid lunch, and a Gatorade with chia during my afternoon workout. Sometimes I'll have a few handfuls of a healthy cereal in the evening, but often that's it for the night. This way I can take one or two nights out a week with friends, have a great dinner, and stay on track. For those of you who prefer three solid meals a day, Phase Three will teach you what foods you can enjoy and still maintain your weight, your energy, and the incredible feeling of good health.

Phase Two is a great first step, during which you learn to choose lunches that won't leave you bloated and tired. You probably won't need an afternoon snack anymore.

You'll be energized enough to return to work for a productive afternoon and enjoy an evening workout that will boost both your mood and your metabolism.

There are countless reasons to exercise—better body, sleep, sex, health, and mood among them. More important, research from the earliest studies of London bus drivers has shown that exercise saves lives and cuts the risk of heart attack and sudden death. This landmark study showed that conductors on London buses had much lower rates of heart attack than bus drivers because they got plenty of exercise climbing up and down the stairs of the double-decker buses, while the drivers sat still for hours in stressful London traffic.

EXERCISE: THE ULTIMATE TOOL IN WEIGHT LOSS

If you think you hate to exercise, get ready to change your mind! You're ready for it now. Your muscle fuel stores are loaded and ready to power amazing workouts. Exercise will no longer be painful or even uncomfortable. Start at a slow pace, one you can manage easily. Your discomfort threshold will rise rapidly so that you'll be exercising harder and harder with no pain. If you're not itching to work out, scale back your pace. Many people push hard every day but have ever-diminishing results. It may seem counterintuitive, but this can be fixed by taking some really, really easy days. You can still burn plenty of calories on low-intensity days by working out longer, and the following days will be pure joy. Remember, if there is any advantage to being overweight, it is that you also have a large muscle mass, and that can BURN calories!

Try to exercise every day, preferably in the afternoon, but morning is fine too. Morning exercise will boost metabolism and speed the awakening of cortisol and thyroid hormones. The only downside to morning exercise is that you're not physiologically at your best, so you won't run, bike, or swim quite as fast as you would later in the day. This is important for really serious athletes, but not too important for weight loss. Morning exercisers are generally more consistent, probably because they get their workouts in before other activities can interfere.

From a performance perspective, afternoon is the best time to exercise. This is when we hit a mental slump just as we're reaching our physiological peak, so working out toward the end of your workday or in the early evening will feel fantastic. Then you can sip a chia smoothie for dinner and enjoy an incredibly good night's sleep.

We've chosen a handful of activities both indoors and out that will feel good and burn lots of calories. Pick a few and switch it up to avoid boredom or injury.

Indoors

First choose a gym. Select one that's affordable and close to home. If you suffer from the so-called Lycra syndrome and feel intimidated by ultra-fit folks strolling the gym, choose a franchise that caters to those new to exercise, such as Anytime Fitness.

Next, get a trainer to show you how to use the equipment and go for the newer machines. There is excellent equipment out now that teaches you the workout patterns of the very fit, helping you burn tons of calories. These machines also guide your body into proper positioning so you have correct technique.

If you haven't been exercising and you're overweight, you may have a huge advantage. You may have a lot of underutilized muscle that can burn a lot of calories. To leverage your muscle mass, choose exercises that use the biggest muscle groups. A big, overweight man doesn't belong on a stationary bike, for example. Using just a small amount of muscle mass on the bike, he may burn 300 calories an hour while sipping a 280-calorie sports drink.

It is much more effective to CLIMB. Climbing utilizes your calves, thighs, buttocks, and even upper body. The more muscles you use, the easier exercise feels because you're spreading the workload over so many muscles. Using a small group of muscles at a high intensity really hurts. Don't do it! You can burn 300 calories an hour on a stationary bike or 1,200 climbing. What a difference! Use an arc trainer or uphill treadmill to climb at 15 degrees.

ARC TRAINER

I love this machine! I use it all winter. It's like the elliptical trainer, but it's kinder to your knees and draws you into a much longer and higher step. This distributes work over your biggest muscles groups, making it feel really easy, but it burns nearly twice as many calories as a regular elliptical! Stair climbers kill my knees, but the Arc Trainer helps them heal.

TREADMILL

Running on a treadmill is about the most boring thing on the planet and hard on your body as well. Instead, increase the pitch to 15 degrees and just walk. Take your iPad, newspapers, magazines, or movies and work or play while you're working out. This is super-easy and burns hundreds of calories. I took a 305-pound friend of mine named Scotty to a hotel gym in Orlando, Florida. Scotty had started eating chia but hadn't exercised in twenty years and avoided it like a bad rash. After three minutes of walking uphill on a treadmill he was sold. "Hey, Doc, I can do this!" he said. And he did, eventually losing dozens of pounds as a result.

ROWING

Rowing burns the greatest number of calories per hour because it engages every major muscle group: calves, thighs, buttocks, lats, abdominals, triceps, biceps, and forearm muscles. Rowing is hard to do continuously, so you may want to do it in increments of a few thousand meters at a time. It will take your body longer to adapt to rowing, so try it a couple of times a week between other types of exercise. Be sure to learn the proper technique to protect your back from injury. (I relate the leg drive to jumping off a diving board.)

IPAD

This bit of equipment is the biggest revolution in exercise because it makes the minutes and hours fly by. You can load up your favorite newspapers, magazines, books, movies, and music. I like to work while working out; I put a rubberized cover on my iPad so it sticks to the sill of the machines, and I use the time to catch up on my reading and emails. I lose no time from work and get a lot done while I'm exercising.

RESISTANCE TRAINING

While aerobic exercise burns more fat, resistance training is necessary to build muscle mass. The more muscle mass you have, the greater your resistance to diabetes, so include some resistance training two or three times per week. You can focus on just a few complex exercises that employ multiple large muscle groups to burn the most calories and gain the most new muscle mass. Squats, pull-ups, and bench presses are the top three. Use machines to help you do these so you can control the resistance.

An eight-month Duke University study published in the *American Journal of Physiology* compared aerobic exercise to weight lifting. "The participants in the aerobic group did the equivalent of 12 miles of jogging per week at 80 percent maximum heart rate, while those in the resistance group did three sets of eight to 12 repetitions three times per week." The study found that aerobic exercise significantly decreased the amount of belly and liver fat because it burned 67 percent more calories.[1]

New research shows that you can do just as well doing *many* reps at a lower weight as *fewer* reps at a higher weight. This is psychologically much easier, and you'll get the same results!

Outdoors

HIKING

At the famous Canyon Ranch resort and spa, hiking is the premier weight-loss activity. Hiking engages all your major muscle groups. Using poles adds an upper-body workout, further distributing the workload to burn more calories and make your workout easier. (Black Diamond has a wonderful line of hiking poles.) It may take you a year to get fit enough to run long distances, but you can take long hikes right away.

MOUNTAIN BIKING

Unbelievably fun and great exercise, mountain biking is not as hard as it sounds. Getting off paved roads and onto dirt paths dramatically increases the safety factor, and the gearing on mountain bikes makes it very easy to pedal even if you're not used to cycling. Rough terrain and hills increase resistance so you don't have to go fast to get a workout. If you find you like mountain biking, don't skimp on a good bike. Consider it an investment in your health. The gears will change smoothly, and it'll feel great ergonomically, enticing you to work out.

ROAD BIKING

There is no better tool to strip off fat than a high-quality road bike. With chia and a road bike you can quickly and painlessly bring your weight down to wherever you want it to be. The key is doing it right. I do a century (100-mile ride) most weekends through the summer and fall. I train using a power meter so I can put out enormous amounts of power over very long periods of time. I ride at a very high cadence, around 95, so there is very little load on my knees. Biking builds elasticity and springiness so you look, act, and feel young. I ride a carbon fiber Serotta with Lightweight carbon fiber wheels. It cost a ton, but it's the best investment I've ever made in my health.

ROLLING TERRAIN

If you don't have mountains in your backyard, try hiking a park or golf course with rolling terrain. Use a little extra push on the hills to give yourself a natural interval workout.

IN-LINE SKATES

If you have the balance and a safe, smooth surface to skate, in-line skating is still a wonderful workout if you're overweight because it neutralizes body weight. Without the pounding effect of running you can push hard and not get sore.

STAND-UP PADDLING

More like playing than exercising, SUP is a fast-growing sport that delivers an aerobic workout with great results for the core and upper body. Give this a shot if you have access to open water. Oceans, lakes, and rivers are all fair game. Take a lesson to learn the Hawaiian technique and you'll soon be motoring through the water, burning a ton of calories, building your balance, and working your abdominal, back, leg, and arm muscles. I put a waterproof GPS on the deck and aim at 6 miles an hour. Get some technique lessons. You'll *fly!*

SOCIALIZE

Socializing is one of the best motivations to exercise. Find a friend to work out with or attend a charity race or ride. Many sports, such as mountain biking, cycling, and cross-country skiing, host big events with a carnival atmosphere that's far more fun than a calorie-packed cocktail party. Have fun with your exercise!

FREQUENTLY ASKED QUESTIONS

Can I eat dinner instead of lunch?

No. The timing of your calorie input is really important. Eating lunch will boost your metabolism to help you burn more calories during the day and fuel your exercise.

Can I still have snacks?

Yes, if you need them, but a well-chosen lunch may keep you full through the afternoon. Don't eat if you're not hungry.

What should I order if I eat out?

Go for vegetables, lean protein—such as chicken, turkey, or fish—and low-CL grains. Restaurant choice can make or break your diet. Go for Japanese or fresh Mexican when possible. Stay away from Italian, Chinese, and steakhouses. Skip the bread and go first for protein. When the waiter first comes over, I say "No bread, and let me get the main course in right away!"

MOVING ON

After six weeks on Phase Two, move on to Phase Three. Again, if you're tempted to quit, move to Phase Three early rather than return to your old eating habits. The incredible premium foods in Phase Three are staples you can stick with for the rest of your life. Get to know them while you're on Phase Two and incorporate them into your lunches. Use recipes from Phase Three in your Phase Two lunches as well. *Bon appétit!*

PHASE III

CHAPTER 7

PHASE III: REAL LIFE, AZTEC STYLE

By now you've been following the Aztec Diet for at least two months. Congratulate yourself on making it through this 60-day challenge! Once you've reached your ideal weight, Phase Three of the Aztec Diet will make sure you stay there. In Phase Three you return to three meals a day; this is both a great reward and the most perilous part of every diet, the point at which many dieters triumph only to rapidly regain their weight. That will not happen to you.

THE PLAN: THREE MEALS A DAY OF AZTEC FOODS

To guide you through these dangerous traps, we're going to introduce you to the best foods of all time. This is the heart of the Aztec Diet: filling and delicious meals made with nutritious foods that you'll love enough to eat for years to come. There is no specified time to move on from Phase Three because it is geared not for weight loss but for maintenance. Consider Phase Three a guide for how you should always eat henceforth.

Phase Three will teach you not only what to eat but also where these amazing foods come from and why they're so good for you. You'll get a heads-up on mistakes to avoid and every bit of information you'll need to make healthy, efficient food choices. Chapter 8, "Premium Foods," teems with tables on every food group, supplying scores on carb load, inflammation, omega-3 fats, and other key nutrients. The information in the tables varies for the different food groups because we've included only the most important scores for each category.

PHASE THREE

HEALTHY EATING FOR LIFE

BREAKFAST: Lean protein such as an egg white frittata or chia smoothie

LUNCH: Vegetables and lean protein such as Asian chicken salad and corn soup

DINNER: Early, light meal such as salmon with kale and quinoa

Use chia smoothies for occasional meal replacements to recover from special occasions or as a regular breakfast.

Add chia to recipes for baked goods, grains, as a substitute for breading meat or fish, or sprinkled over cereal or yogurt.

Now is a good time to retake the questionnaire in the Appendix. Take it again after six months. You probably already know what it will indicate, as you should be feeling fabulous now. The raging inflammation in your body has been doused, so you may find that the symptoms of asthma, arthritis, bowel disease, and headache have diminished. Your cell membranes and neurons are as smooth as silk; the fuel for pain in your body is gone. Your metabolism turns over like a finely tuned engine.

With every marker of chronic disease faded away, you're primed for exercise, which is a key weapon in fighting weight gain. If you haven't already started, you've run out of excuses. Your muscle fuel stores are full. The large sugar swings are gone. Your energy is at an all-time high. For these reasons you won't dread exercise; you'll *love* it. If you never exercise, at least take a brisk afternoon walk across rolling terrain or uphill on a treadmill.

Like exercise, the chia smoothie is a great weapon in your arsenal now. The coming chapters will help you choose great foods for your meals, but you may want to continue using smoothies as meal substitutes at times. If you're not dining with your family or friends, have a smoothie in the evening to avoid burdening your digestive system while you sleep. If you need to recover from a night out at a favorite restaurant, toss back a chia smoothie the next morning. I have my favorite chia smoothie for breakfast almost every morning, and it always jump-starts my day.

Thus armed, you will never be derailed by a wedding, holiday, or night out again. You have finally been freed of the tyranny of food. Your sense of self-control and self-esteem will grow by the day. Now you're able to explore the treasure chest of foods that will continue to improve your life, your well-being, and your outlook on the future. A varied menu will keep you full while allowing a wider array of nutrients to surge through your body, ensuring that you feel terrific.

THE INSPIRATION: AZTEC EDEN

The core foods of this book are descended from the ancient Aztecs because their crops were arguably the best ever grown. A few powerful foods—corn, squash, beans, amaranth, and chia—provided all the Aztecs needed not just to survive but to thrive and prosper. The Aztecs were incredible farmers. Quality soil, ideal climate, and horticultural skill converged in a single time and place to produce these incredibly nutritious crops that brimmed with micronutrients, fiber, omega-3 fatty acids, antioxidants, and phytochemicals. However, the most striking feature of the Aztec crops was the large amount of protein contained in them. Some, such as chia, are complete plant proteins.

To qualify as a complete protein, a food's amino acid score (AAS) must be at least 100. Chia scores 115. Other Aztec crops, such as corn, are nearly complete proteins that the Aztecs easily completed with the addition of lime and beans or amaranth.

In China, by contrast, the dominant grain has long been rice, which has very little protein, few nutrients, and raises the risk of diabetes. America and Europe have depended overwhelmingly on wheat, which is nutritionally bereft compared to the Aztec grains and, in its refined form, has contributed to a staggering worldwide weight gain. Rice and wheat are both high in calories and low in nutrients.

As Americans we tend to think a meal must have meat at its center and at least one starchy side. Traditional grains, however, allowed the Aztecs to live incredibly well with little animal protein. As Bernard R. Ortiz de Montellano,[1] associate professor of science and technology at Wayne State University, wrote: "Customary Aztec diets satisfied ALL nutritional requirements including vitamin and minerals and the quality of the protein was quite good."

This diet gave the Aztecs nearly superhuman endurance and the strength to become the dominant fighting force in the Western Hemisphere, where they established the largest and richest empire. In Spain, France, and England during the sixteenth century, poor nutrition abounded. People were sick, ridden with disease, and suffered short, painful lives. Across the ocean during the same period, the Aztecs were largely free of disease, outpacing all of Europe in food production. Much of this we know from the works of Bernardino de Sahagún, a Franciscan friar, missionary priest, and pioneering ethnographer who spent decades documenting Aztec culture. Given the astonishing range of new sights, sounds, smells, people, and geography he documented, what struck the Spanish most were the new foods.

The Valley of Mexico at that time was one of the premium places in the world to grow food. From two snowcapped volcanic peaks, draped in layers of mist, waters drained into an enormous basin woven with interconnected waterways. Aztec scholar Richard Townsend wrote eloquently in his book *The Aztecs*: "These linked waters and wetlands covered an area of 400 square miles. Abundant aquifers from the Ajusco Sierra supplied the southern lakes, northern wetlands were replenished by lower springs and summer rainfall. All waters flowed into Lake Texcoco. For millennia in their valley and adjacent basins of the central highlands, there was a predictable cycle of birth fruition, death and renewal."

Life in Tenochtitlan, the Aztec capital city, was as ideal as one could imagine, as the surrounding region was nothing short of an agricultural paradise. Highland valleys at various altitudes favored different strains of crops. The Aztecs were close to the tropical fruits of the Pacific and Atlantic Coasts and situated at the intersection of the Northern and Southern Hemispheric agricultural zones. This made the Valley of Mexico one of the premium places on earth for abundant varieties of wild and domesticated edible plants to grow. The volcanic ash increased the fertility of the soil, retained moisture, and enriched crops with an abundance of minerals. At the foot of the volcanoes, the ash lengthened the growing season. The lands were as fertile as the Nile Delta but with far greater diversity of altitudes, soils, weather, and crops.

Just as America would later become a magnet for skilled industrial workers from across Europe and Asia in the early 1900s, the Aztec Empire attracted hunter-gatherers from all across North America. Bringing with them their best crops, tools, and techniques, tribes arrived to share their horticultural knowledge. This migration concentrated the best possible crops on the most magnificent and varied agricultural lands with experienced and knowledgeable farmers. The result was the cultivation of the healthiest, most nutritious foods on earth.

EAT LIKE AN AZTEC

The foods of the Aztec Diet are neither foreign nor obscure. In many ways, the Aztec Diet was the best, the purest, the *original* American diet. Most of what you probably eat at Thanksgiving dinner is Aztec fare!

- Turkey

- Corn bread stuffing

- Squash

- Candied sweet potatoes

- Pumpkin pie

Common Mexican foods also have Aztec origins:

- Avocado

- Tomato

- Pinto beans

- Corn

- Chocolate

As you learn to select foods such as these for your new lifestyle, think of eating as something that needs to be done efficiently. Chances are you've been unintentionally burdening yourself with hundreds of extra calories and dozens of extra grams of fat and sugar every day. The damaging foods that smother you with fat and sugar come with an opportunity cost as well, robbing you of the chance to load up on great micronutrients that protect you from disease and transform your mood. I would venture, if you're like most Americans, that you're calorie overloaded and terribly deprived of basic nutrients. With more efficient eating you can strip away thousands of unneeded calories, hundreds of grams of sugar and fat, while quadrupling the micronutrients that will make you feel the best you ever have.

The Aztecs couldn't have been more efficient. Profiled by Aztec food researcher Sonja Atkinson, the original diet contained:

- few fats and oils

- no refined sugars

- limited red meats

- lots of fruits and veggies

- no wheat

- exceptionally healthy flours such as amaranth

- herbal teas instead of coffee

- no milk or cheese

Some of you may now be saying to yourselves, "That's great for the Aztecs, but I could never give up milk, cheese, wheat, and red meat." That's okay! I'm not asking you to give them up entirely if you don't want to or if you have a house full of picky kids to feed. The Aztec foods are so efficient that you can replace some of the less healthy foods in your family's diet with Aztec counterparts and radically improve your nutrition overnight.

In the following chapters you'll find a host of tools to guide your food choices:

- **Nutrition tables for every food group**

- **A simple substitution chart that will show you how to replace low-quality carbohydrates with Aztec foods**

- **A list of top foods that should take center stage in your diet**

- **A two-week menu of suggested meals to get you started**

- **Recipes for all the meals in the sample menu**

The nutrition tables distinguish foods that were eaten by the Aztecs at the height of their empire and also include foods that hail from other regions but have similarly high nutritional density. These are superfoods we think the Aztecs would choose were they roaming the world today. Foods from the "Best Foods" table will give you the maximum number of nutrients for the least amount of junk. By that I mean the least amount of sugar in grains, fruits, and vegetables and the least amount of fat in proteins. You'll be able to pack your meals with nutrients without the calories that pack on the pounds. In doing so you'll save thousands of calories each week, just by making great choices.

The tables and meals that follow are not exhaustive; the simplicity of the Aztec Diet is one reason I fell in love with it. Research shows that as food choices have expanded, so have our waistlines. To keep you from wandering astray, the AD will return you to basic foods that provide satiety, energy, leanness, and great health. There are plenty of varied recipes you can make with staple foods, without complicated shopping lists. Pore over the next chapter to get acquainted with these premium foods, and dig in!

THE RECAP

Phase Three is not a diet but a maintenance plan, a guide to healthy living for the rest of your life.

Eat three healthy meals a day, focusing on vegetables, fruits, lean protein, and low-CL grains.

Dinner should be the lightest meal of the day.

Use chia smoothies for occasional meal replacements to recover from special occasions or as a regular breakfast.

Add chia to recipes for baked goods, grains, as a substitute for breading meat or fish, or sprinkled over cereal or yogurt.

Exercise daily.

Sleep well!

CHAPTER 8

PREMIUM FOODS

Here lies the heart of the Aztec Diet, a collection of foods that guarantee you will be lean, energetic, and happy for the rest of your life. Turn to these lists again and again until you know exactly which choices will make you look and feel best. I consult them every day!

SCORING FOODS—A REVIEW

As we explain in the Scoring Foods section at the beginning of the book (page xv), we've pored through all the most important scientific databases to identify healthy foods for you. In this section we've created a table for each food group that includes only the scores that are relevant to choosing good foods from that group. Percentage of fat is important in choosing meats, for example, while Whole Food Markets' ANDI scores help you select the most nutritious vegetables. We've done all the work for you so the tables will make choosing foods a cinch. If you'd like to know more about the scoring categories, you can refer back to the Scoring Foods section at the beginning of the book (starting on page xv).

Next you'll find a section on each food group and a table for each. **The best foods are at the top of the tables; scores decrease as you go down. In each table we've highlighted our top choices. These top picks are compiled in a list at the end of the chapter.** The tables offer critical nutrition information at a glance, but each is followed by a closer look at concepts important to that food group. Chapter 9 contains a sample two-week menu using the best Aztec foods, as well as recipes for every meal on the menu.

THE TABLES

PRIORITIZE PROTEIN

Top AD Protein Choices:

- Wild salmon

- Greek yogurt

- Turkey

- Organic chicken

- Grass-fed beef

- Black beans

- Chia

- Quinoa

Every good diet is based on protein. It not only preserves muscle but also acts as a brake to stop you from overeating.

When a Vermont prison studied the satiety of foods, protein came out on top. The prison staff allowed inmates to overeat fat, protein, and carbs. They found that prisoners easily overate carbs and fats but couldn't overeat protein because of this built-in brake.

The Big Texan, a steakhouse in Amarillo, offers diners a free 72-ounce monster steak if they finish it in an hour. If they can't finish it, they have to cough up around $50. Almost everyone ends up parting with 50 bucks because they just can't overeat protein. I tried it when visiting as a guest on the *Oprah Winfrey Show*. I couldn't do it. Neither can you!

If you were to go out to dinner when you're starving, could you eat three bowls of pasta or a whole pizza? Many of us could. But could you have four whole fish? Probably not. Use protein as your friend in weight loss.

Emphasizing protein was the basis of Robert Atkins's enormous success. His diet prescribed large amounts of satiating protein and stripped away most carbohydrates, which causes carb load to plummet. Although Atkins was vilified when he was alive, recent studies have shown that higher-protein diets do work.

A yearlong study of postmenopausal women published in the *Journal of the American Medical Association* compared the success of four diets: Atkins, Zone, Ornish, and LEARN. At year's end the women in the Atkins group had lost the most weight:

- 10 pounds, Atkins

- 6 pounds, LEARN

- 5 pounds, Ornish

- 3½ pounds, Zone

The Atkins group did as well as the others at improving cholesterol levels.

There can always be too much of a good thing, and too much protein can leach calcium from your bones, as several studies have shown.[1] In healthy people, increasing protein intake to 20 to 25 percent of calories can reduce the risk of heart disease if the protein replaces carbohydrates such as white bread, white rice, or sugary drinks. In a 1,200-calorie diet, 25 percent is just 66 grams of protein—not too much—so, try to make protein account for about a quarter of the food you eat.

As you replace junk carbs and dangerous fats with protein, we want you to choose foods that have the maximum amount of protein and the least amount of fat so that your protein isn't loaded with extra calories. The table below shows meats in increasing order of fat percentage, so the most efficient meats top the list. We have highlighted in bold our top most highly recommended choices.

Proteins

MEAT/EGG	AAS	OMEGA-6	CALORIES	FAT (G)	% FAT
Egg white	**145**	**0**	**16**	**0.1**	**3**
Turkey breast, skinless	**145**	**113**	**117**	**0.7**	**5**
Chicken breast, skinless	**136**	**500**	**150**	**4**	**20**
Turkey dark meat, skinless	**145**	**882**	**135**	**4**	**24**
Eye of round beef	**94**	**115**	**143**	**4**	**25**
Top round steak (London broil)	**94**	**170**	**178**	**5**	**27**
Pork tenderloin	**150**	**378**	**102**	**3**	**28**
Pork chops, top loin	**151**	**393**	**120**	**4**	**31**
95% lean ground beef patty (pan)	**85**	**194**	**139**	**5**	**33**
Lamb, cubed for kabobs or stew	**141**	**510**	**190**	**8**	**36**
Bottom round steak	**94**	**212**	**190**	**8**	**36**
Kansas City/New York strip steak	**94**	**178**	**164**	**7**	**36**
Flank steak	94	165	162	6	39
Top sirloin steak/sirloin strip	94	224	180	8	41
Bison, ground, grass-fed	108	266	152	7	43
Chicken, dark meat, skinless	136	1,515	166	8	43
Chicken thigh, skinless	136	1,764	180	10	47
90% lean ground beef patty (pan)	79	252	173	9	47
70% lean ground beef patty	49	297	202	13	59
Lamb, composite cuts	141	833	230	15	60
1 large egg, scrambled	132	1,169	102	7	66
Beef medalions, filet mignon	144	553	281	22	69
Bacon	124	163	453	36	70
Sausage, Italian pork, 1 link (3 oz)	120	2,257	286	23	72
Pork chops, bone-in	141	2,354	291	24	73
Prime rib	144	697	349	30	77
Hot dog, beef, 1 dog	155	463	169	15	81

Note: All values are based on 3-ounce servings unless otherwise noted.

A Closer Look

The best meats are the leanest proteins with the least fat. Obvious winners are skinless turkey and chicken—again, these scores apply to roasted turkey and chicken, not deli cuts. Red meats such as top round, lean ground beef, and eye of the round are surprisingly lean too. The numbers offer a few surprises. While chicken is considered low in fat, it's relatively high in omega-6 fats, while the lean cuts of beef are not. Not all chicken is low fat; dark chicken meat has 1,515 mg of omega-6 and is 43 percent fat!

We included eggs in the meat table for comparison. An inexpensive and fairly efficient form of protein, eggs have relatively low amounts of omega-6 fats and very high protein quality, with a high AAS of 132. Egg whites have staggering numbers: 3 percent fat with only 16 calories and an AAS of 145!

The meats at the bottom of the list are remarkable for having not only staggering percentages of fat and too many omega-6s, but also high levels of inflammation. The worst example? That icon of American barbecues and city street corners: the hot dog. These fatty proteins are also the least filling, so you lose on every front. They won't deliver enough protein to kill your appetite, so you'll be tempted to eat more, and most of what you're eating is fat. So have one on the Fourth of July or at the occasional barbecue, but otherwise go for lean turkey.

> A 2011 Harvard study showed that a high-carbohydrate diet that's also high in animal protein and fat was positively associated with the risk of type II diabetes in men.[2]

Once again, the Aztecs got it right. The chief Aztec animal protein was turkey, which beats every other animal protein, hands down. You could have a burger with 59 percent fat or turkey (roasted, not deli) with just 8 percent! Here's a list of turkey's impressive superlatives:

- Lowest in fat percentage, with one quarter the fat of chicken
- Lowest omega-6 fatty acids, with almost 5 times less than chicken
- Lowest overall fat

- Lowest saturated fat

- Most filling

- Staggering protein quality with 145 AAS

Fish

The health benefits of eating fish cannot be overstated. With staggering amounts of amino acids, fish have phenomenal protein quality as well as tons of omega-3 fatty acids that are good for the brain and heart, and they're highly anti-inflammatory. Toxins, however, can make eating certain fish a risky business. Don't let that scare you away. We've carefully researched the safety recommendations of the Environmental Defense Fund Seafood Health Alert (http://apps.edf.org/page.cfm?tagID=17694). We'll tell you which fish should headline your menu and which ones you should avoid. This is the most spectacular list in the book, with staggering levels of antioxidants, the highest-quality protein, the highest levels of omega-3 fats, and incredibly lean protein. We have highlighted our top ten picks for fish.

Fish

FISH/SHELLFISH	OMEGA-3 (MG)	PROTEIN (G)	ANTI-INFLAMMATION (POSITIVE NUMBER)	AAS	NOTES
Wild Pacific salmon (chinook)	1,820	22	582	148	high in B$_{12}$, selenium
Mackerel (Atlantic) (avoid King mackerel: high in mercury)	1,200	20	510	148	superhigh in B$_{12}$, high in selenium
Trout	1,170	23	210	148	high in B$_{12}$
Canned salmon (red)	1,070	24	390	146	high in B$_{12}$, selenium
Canned anchovies (European) (rinse first: high in sodium), 1 can	950	13	461	148	high in selenium
Black sea bass (fresh)	730	20	334	148	high in selenium
Mussels (blue)	740	20	268	107	superhigh in B$_{12}$, selenium, manganese

FISH/SHELLFISH	OMEGA-3 (MG)	PROTEIN (G)	ANTI-INFLAMMATION (POSITIVE NUMBER)	AAS	NOTES
Oysters (Pacific, raw)	630	8	333	106	superhigh in B_{12}, high in selenium, iron, zinc
Halibut (Pacific)	570	23	75	148	high in selenium
Scallops (bay or sea)	330	20	138	n/a	high in selenium
EAT ONLY OCCASIONALLY					
Shrimp	295	18	98	113	high in dietary cholesterol
Lobster, spiny	454	22	67	113	
Crab (blue)	467	17	172	113	only Alaskan King crab is approved by EDF
Cod (Atlantic)	146	19	69	148	often fried or baked in too much butter
Farmed Atlantic salmon	1,921	19	−184	148	
Swordfish	898	22	307	148	too high in mercury. The EDF says women of childbearing age should not eat
Eel (American, European, conger)	712	20	48	148	too high in mercury and/or PCBs
Bluefin tuna	1,414	25	n/a	148	very high in mercury and PCBs
Yellowfin tuna	264	26	116	148	borderline safe for mercury; limit to once a week.
Canned "albacore" or "white" tuna	808	20	345	148	limited by EDF for mercury content
Canned "light" tuna	239	22	138	148	choose packed in water, not oil
Tilapia	202	22	63	124	Most tilapia sold in the U.S. is imported from Asia or Latin America, where pollution laws can be lax.

Note: These values are based on 3-ounce servings, cooked, unless noted otherwise. All the best fish and shellfish choices are approved for safe consumption four or more times a week.

A Closer Look

A few extra points about the best fish:

- You can't do much better than wild Pacific chinook salmon. This fish has staggering levels of antioxidants, the most omega-3s, and the highest protein quality of fish, meat, or fowl.

- Trout, among the top five healthiest fish, is the only fish that was eaten by the Aztecs.

- Canned salmon is the most economical choice for high-quality fish. The red salmon fished for canning almost always live in the wild, so they're much lower in mercury than canned tuna.

- Generally, wild is better, but farmed mollusks are the most sustainable type of aquaculture and usually have the lowest amount of mercury, which is why blue mussels are relatively high on the fish list.

LOW OMEGA-3 SCORERS:

Not all fish are high in omega-3s. Saltwater fish produce omega-3 fatty acids in response to cold water and use it as insulation. Hawaiian fish live in warm waters, where they're not challenged to make omega-3s. Shellfish live in shallower, warmer waters. You don't have to shy away from these choices because of the low omega-3 scores; many of these fish, such as cod, are good low-fat sources of protein.

LOWEST-RANKED FISH:

- FARMED ATLANTIC SALMON contains higher levels of dioxins and pollutants than wild salmon. It's also remarkably high in omega-6 fats: 566 mg to wild Pacific chinook's 116 mg.

- SWORDFISH is too high in mercury. The EDF says women of childbearing age should never eat this.

- EEL, though common at sushi restaurants, is too high in mercury and/or PCBs. That goes for all types: American, European, conger.

- BLUEFIN TUNA is very high in mercury and PCBs.

- **YELLOWFIN TUNA** is right on the line for safe levels of mercury. Consumption should be limited to once a week.

- **CANNED "CHUNK" AND "ALBACORE" TUNA** are also limited by the EDF for mercury content.

- **CANNED "LIGHT" TUNA** has no recommended limit, but it contains only 239 mg of omega-3s. Consider canned salmon as an alternative. If you're going to eat canned tuna, choose the "light" version packed in water, not oil.

- **TILAPIA**, called the aquatic chicken of the United States and commonly eaten during the summer, is low in omega-3 relative to other fish. Most tilapia sold in the United States is imported from Asia or Latin America, where pollution laws can be lax.

Vegetarian Proteins

Remember that fish and meat aren't the only sources of protein. Every once in a while I'll have a big juicy hamburger in the belief that I haven't been getting enough protein. But here's the thing: The AAS of hamburger (70 percent lean) is only 49 because it's light on the key amino acid tryptophan. Black beans, on the other hand, score 103, surpassing the benchmark (100 AAS) for complete proteins. Bear in mind that the majority of the world lives on a grain-bean combination of complete proteins and has far lower rates of diabetes, obesity, heart disease, stroke, and cancers than Americans. The bottom line is that vegetarian protein can be a much better choice than many meats, containing much-higher-quality protein. See the tables on beans and nuts (page 114 and 124) for scores on vegetarian proteins.

GRAINS: THE ULTIMATE COMFORT FOODS

The most fundamental principle of this book is that we have all been eating the *wrong* grains. First, we went terribly wrong with the low-fat craze. Many of us interpreted the dire edict to eat low-fat diets as permission to embark on all-day carb binges. The USDA advised us to eat six to eleven carb servings a day, more than for any other food group. Carbs are low in fat, we thought, so they must be healthy, right? Wrong. The grains most of us have been eating cause our carb load, and thus our weight, to soar.

Low-carb diets have succeeded because they lower carb load, but Harvard scientists now say slashing carbs altogether is a mistake too; the *right* grains are healthy and we need them. Eat the right grains, and you gain ultimate control over your waistline and your health. This is our top ten list for grains.

Grains/Starches

GRAIN	CARB LOAD	FIBER (G)	PROTEIN (G)	AAS
*Chia, 2 ounces	2	22	8	115
Wheat bran, ½ cup	2	12.5	4.5	76
Bulgur, cooked, ½ cup	6	4	3	54
Whole wheat pasta, cooked, ½ cup	7.5	3	3.5	43
*Quinoa, cooked, ½ cup	9	2.5	4	106
Sprouted wheat bread, 2 slices	10	6	12	n/a
*Corn tortilla, 2	10	4	2	56
*Amaranth, cooked, ½ cup	10.5	2.5	4.5	108
Brown rice, cooked, ½ cup	11	2	2.5	75
*Sweet potato, baked, 1 large	15	8	4	82

*Aztec foods

A Closer Look

Of the top ten grains in the world, the Aztecs had half! With such powerful grains in their diet it's no wonder they dominated the Western Hemisphere; they were the only people with the nutritional support to succeed. Healthy grains like theirs have three critical properties: protein, low carb load, and antioxidants.

1. Protein:

Aztec grains are lean sources of protein with no cholesterol or animal fats, which accounted for the high energy level and leanness of the Aztec warriors, farmers, builders, and laborers. Protein is critical to brain development and muscle retention, as evidenced by the Aztecs' ability to plan and build the greatest metropolis of their time.

Chia and amaranth are complete proteins, with an AAS greater than 100. These beat many varieties of meat.

2. Low carb load:

Aztec grains have extraordinarily low carb loads. Grain comprised more than 80 percent of the Aztec's daily caloric intake, and yet they remained lean because the grains did not spike their blood sugar levels or overwhelm their metabolic systems with sugar. Chia has a carb load as low as 1 for a single scoop (2 tablespoons).

3. Antioxidants:

Some of the Aztec grains have high amounts of healthy omega-3 fats that contain great quantities of antioxidants. The omega-3s are also carriers of phytochemicals and fat-soluble vitamins, which decrease inflammation and lower oxidative stress. Chia has the highest amount of omega-3 fatty acids of any agricultural product on earth. Compare its inflammation score to that of more common grains:

- Wheat flour: −421

- Rice: −153

- Chia: +77

We'd like to see you score 50 or higher for inflammation for an entire day. You can get there with a single serving of chia.

The grains in the preceding table won't tax your body's insulin production or glucose storage capabilities. Their low carb load and high fiber content make them difficult to overeat, unlike Western grains. Because Western grains are almost devoid of fiber and cause wide swings in blood sugar, they wash through the digestive track quickly and leave you wanting more. If you take only a single piece of advice from this book, let it be this: Substitute Aztec grains for products made with refined flours. Even if you make no other changes in your diet, this substitution will be transformative.

Let's compare carb bombs to great Aztec foods. Check these out for yourself at Self Nutrition (http://nutritiondata.self.com) or the University of Sydney's tables (http://www.ncbi.nlm.nih.gov/pmc/articles/PMC2584181/bin/dc08-1239_index.html), two of the easiest food scoring sites to use. The first table contains carb load values for 8 common foods, mostly grains. None of these foods is terribly bad for you individually. If, however, you eat several of them a day, you'll have a sky-high carb load and with it the risk of obesity or even type II diabetes. The second table contains carb load values for several Aztec foods. To maintain your weight (and health!), keep your total carb load under 100 per day. If you're trying to lose weight, keep it under 50 per day.

BOMBS AWAY!

STARCH	CL
Plain bagel, 1 large	33
Macaroni and cheese (boxed), 180 grams	33
French bread, 1 large slice	33
Hard pretzels (enriched flour), 10 twists	32
Russet potato, 150 grams	28
Spaghetti (enriched durum wheat), 1 cup	24
White rice, 1 cup	24
Rice noodles, 1 cup	20
TOTAL	227

MUCH BETTER!

AZTEC FOOD	CL
Chia, 1 ounce	1
Peppers: sweet, red, raw, 1 cup	3
Guacamole, 3 ounces	2
Jícama, 1 cup	2
Cashews, 1 ounce	3

AZTEC FOOD	CL
Corn tortilla, 1	5
Amaranth, 100 grams	9
Sweet corn, 1 ear	9
Black beans, 1 cup	14
Sweet potato, 1 cup	15
TOTAL	63

If one day you ate four foods from the first table—a bagel for breakfast, spaghetti and French bread for lunch, and a stir-fry dinner over white rice—your total carb load would be 114, well over the healthy limit of 100 without snacks or drinks. Eat four Aztec grains instead—chia, sweet corn, a corn tortilla, and amaranth—and your score is just 24. Even if you ate all the foods in the Aztec table in one day, your total carb load would be just 63. It is the difference between these numbers—114 and 24—that will keep you slim and healthy for the rest of your life. The following chart will help you make these substitutions in your everyday meals. When you would ordinarily eat the foods on the left, choose those from the right instead.

SUBSTITUTION CHART

WESTERN FOOD	AZTEC SUBSTITUTION
Bread	Corn tortilla or sprouted whole wheat bread
Rice	Quinoa, amaranth, or bulgur
Potatoes	Sweet potatoes
Breakfast bagel	Chia smoothie, Greek yogurt, or high-fiber cereal
Chips, pretzels, crackers	Mary's Gone Crackers (blend of brown rice, quinoa, flax seeds, and sesame seeds) or kale chips
Pasta (traditional durum wheat)	Quinoa pasta

Breakfast Cereals

America has had a love affair with grains since the birth of breakfast cereals in the nineteenth century. John Harvey Kellogg, a doctor, launched the grain-for-breakfast revolution in the 1890s when he introduced cereals that would replace bacon and eggs for the rich and gruel for the poor.

Although we've been advising you to avoid most Western grains, cereal is a great source of soluble fiber—especially if I can't sell you on beans or large quantities of vegetables. Soluble fiber helps you stay full, control weight, and stave off diabetes. Harvard's School of Public Health recommends that women ages 19–50 consume 25 grams of fiber per day, men ages 19–50 should consume 38 grams per day. While cereal is a great source of fiber, some brands have very high carb loads. Even in the best cereals CL jumps from 7 to 17. The following table will help you choose cereals that will deliver major fiber for very few calories and avoid the ones that will steal your whole CL quota for the day.

Cereals

CEREAL	CL	ANTI-INFLAMMATION (POSITIVE NUMBER)	FIBER (G)	CALORIES
Kellogg's Special K Protein Plus	7	8	7	134
Quaker Puffed Wheat	7	−32	1	55
Kashi GOLEAN regular	11	−78	10	148
Fiber One Original	12	−20	28	120
General Mills Cheerios (plain)	12	−10	3	103
General Mills Kix	12	−35	2	88
Oatmeal, regular, cooked	14	−96	4	166
Uncle Sam cereal	15	13	13	237
Nature's Path Optimum Slim	16	−97	11	180
Kashi GOLEAN Crunch!	17	−103	8	200
Cornflakes	17	−100	1	101
Raisin bran	26	−156	7	190
Frosted mini wheats	29	−188	6	203

Note: All values are based on 1-cup servings.

CEREAL	CL	ANTI-INFLAMMATION (POSITIVE NUMBER)	FIBER (G)	CALORIES
Muesli	41	−232	6	289
Low-fat fruit granola	44	−303	5	318
Low-fat granola w/raisins	47	−198	6	345
Grape-nuts	56	−274	10	416

A Closer Look

Some of the best cereals, such as Fiber One and Kashi GOLEAN, are astounding sources of dietary fiber, especially given how few calories they have. Cereals like these put extra fiber in your diet and can make a great breakfast or snack with almond milk.

The cereals in the bottom half of the table quickly climb in carb load and calories, and they're also more inflammatory. I love Grape-nuts, but the carb load in one cup is as much as we recommend in a whole day if you're trying to lose weight, so I eat only a half cup. The granolas and muesli, though commonly perceived as health foods, are high in calories and carb load and are comparatively low in fiber. I find that just a single high-carb-load meal can throw off my whole day.

DAIRY

Two key nutrients in the Aztec Diet are protein and calcium. You should be getting protein from fish, meats, beans, nuts, and some grains, so for dairy we focus on getting plenty of calcium, which dieters often lose, with the lowest number of calories and carb load. We've scored dairy products and dairy substitutes for calcium, carb load, protein, and calories. You'll see that yogurt with fruit mixed in carries half a day's carb load, while skim milk, almond milk, soy milk, and goat's milk give you a good dose of calcium without a ton of calories or a high carb load.

Dairy

FOOD	CALCIUM (MG)	CL	PROTEIN (G)	CALORIES
Almond milk, unsweetened, 1 cup	200	0	1	40
So Delicious coconut milk, unsweetened, 1 cup	100	0	1	50
Part-skim mozzarella, ¼ cup shredded	200	1	7	85
American cheese, ¼ cup diced	193	1	8	131
Blue cheese, ¼ cup crumbled	178	1	7	120
Light string cheese, 1 piece	150	1	6	50
Low-fat Cheddar or Colby, ¼ cup diced	137	1	8	57
Cream cheese, 2 tablespoons	28	1	2	100
Hemp milk, 1 cup	20	5	5	110
Nonfat cottage cheese, 1 cup	125	6	15	104
Goat's milk, 1 cup	327	8	9	168
Nonfat Greek yogurt, plain, 1 cup	250	8	20	120
Skim milk, 1 cup	300	9	8	80
2% milk, 1 cup	286	9	8	122
Soy milk, 1 cup	60.7	9	8	131
Nonfat plain yogurt, 1 cup	488	11	14	137
Soy yogurt (Silk, plain), 1 container	300	11	6	150
Rice milk, enriched original, 1 cup	300	17	1	120
Nonfat fruit yogurt, 1 cup	372	24	11	233

Note: If you're a vegetarian or vegan, as many readers are, you can easily increase your calcium consumption by adding almond milk to your diet.

The Institute of Medicine recommends daily calcium intake by age group as follows:

AGE	CALCIUM MG/DAY
0–6 mo.	200
7–12 mo.	260
1–3	700
4–8	1,000
9–18	1,300

AGE	CALCIUM MG/DAY
19–50	1,000
51–70 (male)	1,000
51–70 (female)	1,200
71+	1,200

Depending on your age and diet, you may have to work to get enough calcium with multiple servings. Chia and vegetables such as kale (93 mg per cup) and spinach (245 mg per cup!) are great sources of calcium.

BEANS AND LEGUMES

Beans are one of the world's greatest nutritional gems. They have staggering amounts of soluble fiber and a moderate carb load; they are high in protein, filled with micronutrients, and excellent for quelling hunger. Beans do cause gas because they contain a sugar called *raffinose*, which creates gas pockets in the large intestine as they're digested. But don't worry; I like to call gas a passing problem! That's because it does go away with the right steps. Here are several ways around it:

■ Adaptation: After several weeks on the AD the bad gut bacteria will be washed out and you'll have new, healthier gut bacteria, making you less prone to gas.

■ Soaking beans (fresh, not canned) overnight cuts down their gas levels significantly.

■ Cooking with bay leaf, fennel, cilantro, turmeric, rosemary, or anise also reduces gas levels.

■ If you're really taxed, take Beano!

We have a lot of information to share about beans and legumes. The table offers a glance at the most salient scores. All beans rate high in fullness and nutrient density, for example, so those scores are not included. The most remarkable thing about beans is how many of them are complete proteins with AAS values over 100. Following the table you'll find tips about complementary proteins and additional nutrients.

LEGUMES

LEGUME	AAS	CL	ANTI-INFLAMMATION	FIBER (G)	PROTEIN (G)
Black-eyed peas	116	13	−22	11	13
Garbanzo beans	107	23	−127	11	12
Refried	106	13	−72	12	13
Tofu (raw)	106	2	−16	0	10
Great Northern	104	13	−53	12	15
*Black	103	14	−45	15	15
Split peas	102	13	−67	16	16
Soybeans (edamame)	93	6	64	8	17
Navy	91	15	−48	19	15
Pinto	89	15	−40	15	15
Kidney	89	15	−55	11	15
Lentils	86	13	−15	16	18
Green peas	84	9	−6	9	9
Fava beans	84	13	−53	9	13
Baked beans (vegetarian)	71	19	−103	10	12
Tempeh (fermented bean curd)	n/a	1	−14	0	5

*Aztec foods

Note: All values are based on 1 cup of fresh (not canned), cooked, unsalted beans, unless noted otherwise. CL does not change much between canned and cooked.

A Closer Look

■ BLACK BEANS are high in folate, iron, and magnesium. Just 1 cup delivers 30 percent of your daily protein requirement in an incredibly lean 227 calories. Try black bean soup!

■ PINTO BEANS are high in folate, iron, magnesium, and potassium. Complementary proteins (which combine with a food to render the dish a complete protein of 100 AAS or higher) are corn, nonfat yogurt, barley, bulgur, wheat flour, cornmeal, millet, kamut, buckwheat, brown rice, and amaranth.

- **KIDNEY BEANS:** Complementary proteins are corn, nonfat yogurt, wheat flour, cornmeal, bulgur, buckwheat, and spelt. An extract of white kidney beans was shown to block the absorption of carbs and aid in weight loss.[3]

- **GREAT NORTHERN BEANS** are high in folate, magnesium, potassium, and iron.

- **NAVY BEANS** are high in folate, iron, magnesium, and potassium. Complementary proteins are salmon, corn, wheat flour, oats, spelt, bulgur, and cornmeal.

- **REFRIED BEANS** are high in vitamin C, iron, magnesium, and potassium. I always avoided refried beans because I assumed they were fried twice! In fact, the good ones aren't fried at all. The bad ones are cooked with lard and can be packed with sodium, as much as 600 mg. But the good ones are pure heaven. Try Amy's Vegetarian Organic refried beans, which are low in salt and contain organic onions and spices.

- **GREEN PEAS:** Yes, they're a legume and high in vitamins C, K, and A. The omega ratio is higher than some, but the omega-6 count is low. Complementary proteins are fish, corn, wheat flour, oats, and cornmeal.

- **LENTILS** are high in folate, iron, and potassium. Complementary proteins are fish, corn, wheat flour, oats, and cornmeal. Many studies link lentils, especially their fiber, to weight loss. Here's just one round-up from Discovery: http://health.howstuffworks.com/wellness/food-nutrition/natural-foods/natural-weight-loss-food-lentils-ga.htm.

- **BLACK-EYED PEAS** rank the highest of all beans in protein quality, with an AAS of 116. They are also high in vitamins K and A, folate, calcium, iron, and potassium.

- **SPLIT PEAS** are high in folate and potassium. Their omega-6 count is low, so they're a fine choice.

- **GARBANZO BEANS** have the highest omega-6 count of all beans, clocking in with an astonishing 10,932. Choose another bean.

- **BAKED BEANS** are not complete proteins, and even the vegetarian variety has 20 grams of sugar. Substitute kidney beans.

VEGETABLES

If you already had a diet rich in vegetables you probably wouldn't be reading this book. I'm not a big veggie lover myself, so I'm not going to try too hard to sell you on vegetables. Instead, I recommend adding to your diet a few premium vegetables that are chock-full of nutrients and forgoing the rest. Some vegetables are worthless to dieters because they're low in nutrients and fullness factor, and you may have to douse them in omega-6 fats to eat them. Kale, collard greens, and watercress, on the other hand, earn a perfect ANDI score of 1,000 for a single serving. I hide these in my morning shake for staggering nutrient levels with no vegetable taste. Their carb load scores are super low. Their anti-inflammatory scores are the highest imaginable . . . 462 for kale and 466 for spinach! We've included in the table only vegetables that are high in fullness and nutrient density, so those scores are not included.

Vegetables

VEGETABLE	ANDI	CL	ANTI-INFLAMMATION
Kale, cooked, 1 cup	1,000	4	462
Collards, cooked, 1 cup	1,000	4	379
Watercress, raw, 1 cup	1,000	0	36
Spinach, cooked, 1 cup	739	2	466
Cabbage, Napa, 1 cup	704	2	23
Brussels sprouts, cooked, 1 sprout	672	1	12
Arugula, raw, 1 cup	559	0	1
Red or green leaf lettuce, raw, 1 cup	406	1	48
Broccoli, cooked, 1 stalk	376	5	143
*Pumpkin, canned, 1 cup	372	6	334
Red pepper, sweet, raw, 1 cup	366	3	126
*Tomatoes, red, raw, 1 cup	190	2	17
*Squash, summer, cooked, 1 cup	136	3	2
Iceberg lettuce, 1 cup	110	1	7
*Onion, raw, 1 cup	50	5	374

*Aztec foods

A Closer Look

Exposed to only 2 percent of the world's land mass, the Aztecs cultivated four of the top vegetables, once again showing the quality nutrients that their rich, black soil allowed them to grow, as well as their uncanny ability to pick winning foods.

This table helps you pick veggies that count. If you're making a salad, for example, use arugula, watercress, or spinach instead of iceberg for a major upgrade in nutrients. A quick, delicious Aztec snack for those of you who never eat veggies: pico de gallo. Just toss together tomatoes, onions, jalapeño, cilantro, and a little lime juice.

If you're like me and don't like limp, soggy cooked veggies, leave them raw and crisp. Or disguise them in your chia smoothie. Barbara Rolls, an amazing researcher and scientist at Penn State, showed that children and adults ate significantly more vegetables if they were hidden in a puree. Soups are another wonderful vehicle for veggies. The vegetables take on the flavor of the soup and add lovely texture. Soups also aid weight loss. Having vegetable soup as a first course has proved to be a highly effective strategy to reduce the intake of higher-calorie foods during a meal.

Some of the least nutritious vegetables include iceberg lettuce (devoid of nutrients and almost always slathered with fattening salad dressing), water chestnuts (nutrient devoid), and canned vegetables of all kinds, which contain too much sodium and may have traces of BPA leached from cans.

FRUITS

Perfect, whole foods, fruits are excellent, satisfying treats. We love them whole or blended into chia smoothies. Like soups, they've been shown to reduce energy intake when eaten at the start of a meal. As good as fruits are, however, their nutrient content pales in comparison to veggies. Look at the ANDI ratings. The top vegetables score 1,000, whereas cranberries, one of the top-ranked fruits, score just 236. Fruits still have many benefits, though. Consumption of anthocyanin-rich foods, particularly blueberries, can decrease the risk of type II diabetes.[4] The following fruits all have high fullness values, so we've included only scores for ANDI, carb load, and anti-inflammation power. I use frozen Maine wild blueberries in my chia smoothies for a higher antioxidant boost.

Fruits

FRUIT	ANDI	CL	ANTI-INFLAMMATION (POSITIVE NUMBER)
Cranberries	236	2	−4
*Guava	223	7	131
Strawberries	212	3	28
Blackberries	178	4	6
Raspberries	145	3	1
Lemon	141	4	19
Blueberries	130	6	−16
*Papaya	118	3	33
Orange	109	6	9
Grapefruit	102	4	13
*Cantaloupe	100	5	76
*Starfruit	100	3	4
Lime	99	1	2
Watermelon	91	3	−7
*Pineapple	64	6	65
Bananas	30	18	−115
Apple	2	3	−21

*Aztec

Note: All information is for raw fruit. All values are based on one-cup servings.

A Closer Look

Stay away from dried fruit and fruit juice.

- DRIED FRUITS have sky-high CLs due to the concentration of sugar. Raisins, for example, have a CL of 75!

- FRUIT JUICES carry high CLs and low ANDI scores and aren't filling. Drink water and eat whole fruit.

FATS

Fats are highly satisfying foods that stave off hunger and delay stomach emptying, so they're not all to be avoided. The AD recommends two kinds of fats: omega-3s and omega-9s. You'll get plenty of other fats in your diet without trying—saturated fats in certain dairy products and meats, omega-6s in vegetable oils and nuts—so focus on adding omega-3s and omega-9s and cutting down on omega-6s. Omega-6 fats are found in the vegetable oils commonly used in food manufacturing and cooking, as well as in salad dressings.

Good Fats

OMEGA-3 FATS

These beneficial fatty acids fall into two categories, marine and plant. Marine sources include fish and fish oils, and their chief advantage is one called *DHA*, which crosses the blood-brain barrier, so it improves the quality of neurons in the brain. They have been used successfully to treat depression and bipolar disease. Another fish oil, called *EPA*, has countless heart benefits, including prevention of arrhythmias, congestive heart failure, and heart attack.

Consult the fish chart (pages 102–3) to see which fish have the highest concentrations of omega-3s and avoid those contaminated with mercury. When shopping for fish oils, look for molecularly distilled oils that have taken out any heavy metal contamination. Look for brands that have 60 percent more EPA than DHA. Check our section on supplements in the Appendix for suggested brands. I buy mine from my local pharmacist to be certain I'm getting a high-grade fish oil. Www.consumerlab.com has an excellent review of all available brands. I've used Nordic Naturals and Solgar's fish oil products. The key is that they are molecularly distilled and have no heavy metals.

Fish oils have a range of effects on heart disease. Here are some recent studies:

- One of my favorite heart researchers, Eric Rimm, ScD, of Harvard's School of Public Health, published an August 2011 study showing that older adults with high levels of EPA had a 50 percent lower incidence of congestive heart failure.[5]

- A Danish study showed an increased risk of heart disease in women of reproductive age who took little or no fish oil.[6]

- An English study showed a modest decrease in blood pressure with fish oil supplements.[7]

- A U.S. Environmental Protection Agency study showed omega-3 fatty acid supplements offer protection against the adverse cardiac and lipid effects associated with air pollution exposure.[8]

- A Harvard study showed that circulating fish oils can decrease the risk of atrial fibrillation, a very common heart rhythm irregularity found in older Americans. Without blood-thinning therapy, this can become fatal.[9]

The top plant-based sources of omega-3s are:

- Chia

- Flax

- Nuts and seeds

- Spirulina or chlorella, types of algae

Chia contains the highest plant concentration of omega-3s and is one of the few suppliers of the omega-3 ALA. Algae is a terrific source of omega-3s for those who are concerned about overfishing. Most algae supplements contain primarily EPA, but there are some newer formulas with a balance of EPA and DHA.

Harvard's Walter Willett offered the best advice for getting omega-3s into your diet: Eat fish several times a week and a daily serving of plant-based omega-3s. This helps bring you closer to the ideal 3:1 ratio of omega-6 to omega 3 fats and improves the health of your heart and brain. Two servings of wild salmon a week and two scoops of chia a day will do the trick!

OMEGA-9 FATS

The omega-9s found in olive oil are incredibly heart-healthy fats with a long history of enriching diets. Neolithic people used olive oil as long ago as 8,000 B.C. Homer called it liquid gold. Olive oil is the core of the lauded Mediterranean diet. It became the first health fad and remains a top-rated food today. There is a much lower incidence of heart attack and stroke in areas where olive oil is consumed daily. Here are just a few of the reasons why:

- Olive oil lowers bad (LDL) cholesterol and, more significantly, raises good (HDL) cholesterol.

- Hydroxytyrosol, the main antioxidant compound in olives, is tremendously anti-inflammatory.

- Olive oil can help decrease blood pressure and the likelihood of clotting.

- Olive oil is loaded with the polyphenols oleuropein and tyrosol. These help arteries become more elastic so they are pliant and resistant to stress.

- Olive oil is the single ingredient in the Mediterranean diet that is likely responsible for improved brain health and decreased blood clots in the brain, as detected by CT scan.

You don't need a lot of olive oil. Former president of the American Heart Association Scott Grundy says that the difference between a high-fat and low-fat diet lies in just 2 tablespoons of olive oil. Eat more than that and you're well over budget for fats. Use olive oil for cooking or salad dressings. Just whisk with balsamic vinegar or fresh lemon juice and salt and pepper.

Fats to Limit

SATURATED FATS (—BAD!)

Saturated fats, found in whole dairy products and fatty red meats, are devoid of healthy vitamins and antioxidants. Like trans fats, they increase cholesterol levels, and they make people fat! Each gram of carbohydrate or protein has 4.5 calories, but saturated fat packs in a walloping 9 calories per gram. Follow the AD food recommendations and you'll largely avoid them.

TRANS FATS (—ULTRA BAD)

These are used in many processed foods to add texture and improve shelf life and crispness. They are more harmful than naturally occurring oils. They lower the good cholesterol and raise the bad cholesterol to increase your risk of heart disease. There is no requirement for this in the diet.

OMEGA-6 FATS (—LIMIT)

Decades ago heart doctors determined that omega-6 fats are better for the heart than saturated fats. This is true. However, omega-6 fats don't have the health benefits of omega-3s and omega-9s, and they can increase pain in your body.

Having more omega-6s in your diet means more omega-6 in the membranes of your body's cells. This prompts the cells to produce inflammatory messenger hormones that send signals to other cells to increase the amplitude of pain in sensory nerves. In breast cancer survivors with high amounts of omega-6s, breast duct cells are more inflamed and hyperresponsive to estrogen. Omega-3 fats tend to calm these cells down. This discovery prompted a nutrition school dean to remark that in switching from saturated fats to polyunsaturated fats we sacrificed women's breasts for men's hearts. Better to avoid both! I stay away from vegetable oils, with the exception of olive oil, to avoid the problem. Olive oil should be your only significant source of omega-6. The better fats are in bold type in the following table.

Fats

OIL/FAT	ANTI-INFLAMMATION (POSITIVE NUMBER)	OMEGA-6	OMEGA-3
Flaxseed oil, 1 tablespoon	**142**	**1,715**	**7,196**
Olive oil, 1 tablespoon	**71**	**1,318**	**103**
Canola oil, 1 tablespoon	**56**	**3,217**	**812**
Almond butter, 2 tablespoons	**38**	**3,802**	**134**

OIL/FAT	ANTI-INFLAMMATION (POSITIVE NUMBER)	OMEGA-6	OMEGA-3
Peanut butter, 2 tablespoons	18	4,709	27
Peanut oil, 1 tablespoon	−3	4,321	n/a
Regular margarine, 1 tablespoon	−11	3,128	275
Mayonnaise, 1 tablespoon	−18	2,320	290
Soybean oil, 1 tablespoon	−36	6,807	917
Butter, unsalted, 1 tablespoon	**−44**	**382**	**44**
Corn oil, 1 tablespoon	−49	7,224	157
Coconut oil, 1 tablespoon	−111	243	trace

A Closer Look

Flaxseed oil, olive oil, almond butter, and canola oil are all good anti-inflammatory oils that offer a whole days' dose of antioxidants in a single serving. Minimize use of the inflammatory fats and pay attention to those high in omega-6 fats. Flaxseed and canola oils boast the most favorable ratios. Almond butter, although it's anti-inflammatory, corn oil, and peanut butter have appalling omega-6:omega-3 ratios.

Next, look at the amount of omega-6 in a fat to see what it'll do to your daily consumption. Butter is a reasonable choice if you're not watching your cholesterol. You don't want to eat gobs of it—one pat a day will do—but it's preferable to margarine, which contains eight times as many omega-6 fats. Soybean oil, corn oil, and peanut butter slam you with more than your entire daily consumption.

The National Institutes of Health reports that a low ratio of omega-6 fats to omega-3 fats reduces the incidence and symptoms of heart disease, breast cancer, rheumatoid arthritis, asthma, and colorectal cancer.[10]

Most vegetable oils have more fat per tablespoon than is found in a serving of many kinds of beef. The simplest approach is to avoid them, especially for cooking and salad dressings. I'd rather eat a serving of kale or sweet potato than a salad, anyway, as many salads have fewer nutrients than one superveggie. Having to pour 8 grams of fat on the salad becomes pretty counterproductive!

NUTS AND SEEDS

Nuts were a crucial source of protein for the Aztecs. As you can see in the following table, the top four nuts score as well as or better than many meats do for protein quality. Most nuts are anti-inflammatory, so they can significantly boost your daily inflammation score. Brazil nuts, macadamia nuts, and ground flaxseeds, in particular, are packed with antioxidants. The only disadvantage of nuts is that they're high in omega-6 fats (except macadamia nuts), so keep portions small. The nuts and seeds in bold type in the following table have the highest protein quality.

Nuts/Seeds

NUT/SEED (1 OUNCE)	AAS	ANTI-INFLAMMATION (POSITIVE NUMBER)	OMEGA-6
*Pumpkin and squash seeds	**136**	**−24**	**5,326**
Pistachios	**109**	**17**	**3,729**
Cashews	**100**	**13**	**2,179**
Flaxseeds, ground	**92**	**137**	**1,655**
Sunflower seeds	81	−40	9,180
Peanuts	70	24	4,355
Brazil nuts	67	175	5,758
Almond butter (2 tablespoons)	66	76	3,802
Peanut butter (2 tablespoons)	55	18	4,709
Walnuts	55	−38	10,761
Almonds	**54**	**54**	**3,378**
Macadamia nuts	4	133	366

*Aztec foods

BEVERAGES

A solid beverage plan is a vastly underrated tool for weight control. Beverages can help maintain weight by filling you up, diminishing hunger, and reducing the number of calories eaten at meals. Or they can be downright villainous, adding hundreds of extra calories and spiking your daily carb load. The best beverage choices are highlighted in bold type in the following table.

Harvard's Eric Rimm concluded that the link between artificially sweetened beverages and type II diabetes is largely explained by failing to control health status, dieting, and body mass index for other variables.[11]

Beverages

BEVERAGE (1 CUP)	CALORIES	CL
Almond milk, unsweetened	40	0
Coconut water	46	3
Tomato juice	49	4
Vegetable juice (V8)	51	4
Skim milk	86	9
Carrot juice	94	8
Grapefruit juice (pink)	96	7
Hemp milk	110	5
Orange juice	112	9
Apple juice	114	6
Rice milk	120	17
Soy milk	131	9
Pomegranate juice	134	8
Cranberry juice cocktail	137	8

A Closer Look

Milks can be good low-calorie sources of both protein and calcium. I pour almond milk on my cereal because it has far fewer calories and a lower carb load than skim milk. Soy milk has more calories and a higher carb load, but it also has more protein. Rice milk sounds healthy, but it's high in calories, low in protein, with nearly double the carb load of cow's and soy milk. Not a good choice! Organic skim cow's milk remains a good source of calcium and vitamin D, and some brands add DHA. If you've been drinking whole or 2 percent milk, switching to skim is one of the easiest, most effective dietary changes you can make. If you drink milk only for calcium, know that there are better sources, such as kale and chia.

A landmark study[12] reported that adolescents who drank milk were leaner in adulthood than those who didn't.

Manufactured vegetable juices aren't as good as they seem. Regular V8 has 600 mg of sodium in an 11.5-ounce can, and there aren't many veggies in it. CSPI reports that a cup of carrot juice has 900 percent of the daily recommended value of vitamin A, while V8 has just 15 percent. Low-sodium V8 works well as a smoothie mixer as long as you add real veggies to it. V8 V-Fusion seems like a terrific concept, but in truth it contains mostly grape and apple juice. The bottom line is that you're better off mixing your own juices and smoothies.

Coca-Cola is my biggest treat in life. I've drunk Coke nearly every day since the beginning of first grade. It's a great reward for me and makes my day. However, I drink only a 6-ounce serving. At that serving size the carb load is only 6, less than that of many of the healthy foods or beverages in the chart. I emphasize having a Coke as a treat or reward for a healthy diet, which is what I do. My carb load for a whole day is only 50, and that includes my 6-ounce Coke. I also use Coke as fuel in bike racing, as do many Tour de France riders.

Coffee and tea are good low-calorie beverages. I start my day with green tea because it gives a smooth energy boost that beats the jumpy kick of highly caffeinated soft drinks and coffees. It's also been reported to help prevent stroke, prostate cancer, and breast cancer. If you prefer coffee, beware of fatty, high-calorie coffee drinks and add-ins. If you need a caffeinated beverage several times a day, black coffee is a good no-calorie alternative to soft drinks. The replacement of one serving of sugar-sweetened beverage with one cup of coffee is associated with a 70 percent reduced risk of type II diabetes.

Water is a grossly underrated, highly effective diet tool. Drink an 8-ounce glass before every meal and two hours afterward. If you eat snacks, drink water with them. Sparkling water with a wedge of lemon or lime is a wonderful soda substitution. Check the sodium content on sparkling waters and club soda. You can also make your own healthy sodas by adding small amounts of pure fruit juice to sparkling water. It's less sweet with a crisper taste.

Fruit juices often contain added sugar, so stick to 100 percent juice and avoid cock-tails, juice drinks, and fruit punch. Orange and grapefruit juices have more nutrients than apple or grape. Portions should be kept small. While fruit juices have more calo-ries and sugar than we recommend, it's okay to use them in chia smoothies if they allow you to add veggies you wouldn't otherwise eat. Juice may add 100 extra calories, but you'll still lose weight and benefit from nutritious vegetables.

TREATS

My friends will tell you I'm the ultimate junk food addict. I *love* my treats. My favorites are Coca-Cola and Scores chocolate bars. People look at me aghast and say, "How can you eat *that*?" I happily explain that my overall meal plan gives me a very low carb load, so the addition of an occasional treat makes very little difference. Sure, soft drinks can cause tremendous weight gain if you guzzle 32 ounces on top of fries and a burger, but a 6-ounce serving now and then will not derail a healthy diet. I believe you should have some reasonable reward to look forward to. Added to a well-planned meal, they're a tiny speed bump in your carb load.

Chocolate is an authentic Aztec food you probably already love, and it's good for you! A review in the *American Journal of Clinical Nutrition* of forty-two studies showed consistent acute and chronic benefits of chocolate or cocoa on flow mediated dilation of blood vessels.[13] The key ingredient appears to be cocoa flavan-3-ols. I enjoy a hot choco-late several times a day. I also eat small chocolate squares, which are low in calories but high in cocoa. That's the good news. The bad news is that you should avoid high-fat, high-sugar chocolates.

SUMMARY

Use the lists in this chapter every day to make great food choices. I keep them on my phone for easy reference when shopping or eating out. We've used these lists to construct whole meal plans that incorporate all the Aztec Diet principles. The meals and recipes you'll find in the next chapter have low carb loads, low inflammation scores, lots of protein, and a good dose of omega-3 fats. You may occasionally eat a high-CL grain since its effect will be balanced by other low-CL foods on the AD. Between meals you'll feel energetic and calm, free of the highs and lows caused by druglike, trashy foods. Constructing these premium food tables has had the greatest effect on my diet of anything I've ever written. Look closely and you'll see that these are very select foods that can deliver a nutritional wallop while helping you stay trim.

Following is our ultimate "Best Foods" list. Here you'll find the top ten foods from each group (except for a few categories in which there aren't that many great choices!). I eat just a few foods from this list and have never felt better! Carry this list around with you. You'll be amazed at how much your nutrition improves.

BEST FOODS

MEAT

Turkey breast, skinless

Chicken breast, skinless

Turkey dark meat, skinless

Eye of round beef

Top round steak (London broil)

Pork tenderloin

Pork chops, top loin

95% lean ground beef

Lamb, cubed for kabobs or stew

Bottom round or New York strip steak

FISH

Wild Pacific salmon

Canned European anchovies

Atlantic mackerel

Trout

Canned red salmon

Black sea bass

Blue mussels

Pacific oysters

Pacific halibut

Bay or sea scallops

GRAINS/STARCHES

Chia

Quinoa

Corn tortillas

Sweet corn

Amaranth

Bulgur

Sprouted wheat bread

Sweet potato

Quinoa pasta

Whole wheat pasta

CEREALS

Kellogg's Special K Protein Plus

Quaker Puffed Wheat

Kashi GOLEAN regular

Fiber One Original

General Mills Cheerios regular

General Mills Kix

Oatmeal, regular

Uncle Sam cereal

Nature's Path Optimum Slim

Kashi GOLEAN Crunch

DAIRY

Almond milk, unsweetened

Coconut milk, unsweetened

Skim cow's milk

Nonfat Greek yogurt, plain

Part-skim mozzarella

Low-fat Cheddar or Colby

BEANS/LEGUMES

Black beans

Kidney beans

Pinto beans

Great Northern beans

Refried beans

Black-eyed peas

Green peas

Lentils

VEGGIES *(any veggie is a good choice, but these are the most nutritious)*

Kale

Collard greens

Watercress

Spinach

Brussels sprouts

Arugula

Napa cabbage

Red or green leaf lettuce

Tomatoes

Onions

FRUITS *(any fruit is a good choice, but these are the most nutritious)*

Grapefruit

Lemon

Lime

Blackberries

Strawberries

Blueberries

Cranberries

Papaya

Orange

Cantaloupe

FATS

Olive oil

Flaxseed oil

Canola oil

Almond butter

Butter

NUTS/SEEDS

Pumpkin and squash seeds

Pistachios

Cashews

Flaxseeds, ground

BEVERAGES

Water

Almond milk, unsweetened

Freshly blended vegetable juice

Coconut water

Skim milk

TREATS

Coke, 6 ounces

Dark chocolate

CHAPTER 9

MEALS AND RECIPES

In this chapter we offer a selection of menus and recipes for breakfast, lunch, and dinner that will carry you through two weeks of Phase Three. By then, you'll hopefully have a handful of new favorite dishes and a whole new take on eating.

Once you move on to selecting foods on your own, be mindful of portion sizes. Eat as many vegetables as you like, but be moderate with all other foods and even beverages. This is make-or-break for many people. Penn State's Barbara Rolls found that a 50 percent increase in food portions resulted in an increase of 423 calories a day in both men and women. A 50 percent increase in the portion of beverages increased calories by 10 percent for women and 26 percent for men.

What you eat is just as important as how much. We've compared nutrition scores for a few meal choices to give a sense of the vast range between healthy and not-so-healthy meals. (Once you've seen the numbers, fast food quickly begins to look like disease in a paper bag.) Compare the scores of the meals that follow. Many will shock you and may quickly reveal the glaring errors in your former diet.

MEAL COMPARISONS

With only 314 calories, my favorite smoothie earns a whopping ANDI score of 3,228 and an incredible anti-inflammation score of 832. That's a whole week's worth of anti-oxidants in one meal! This is how the AD douses the fire inside, and it's why people feel so well that they're rarely tempted to go back to their old eating habits for long. You'll also see how incredibly efficient Aztec eating is. For example, you get an ANDI score of 10 per calorie in the chia smoothie, but only .01 in the All-American meal (burger, fries, and a cola). In other words, you'd have to eat more than 100 All-Americans to get the same nutrients as in a single chia smoothie. No wonder we have a problem with obesity!

> Foods with positive inflammation scores are anti-inflammatory. Foods with negative inflammation scores create inflammation in the body.

Dr. Bob's Kale Blueberry Smoothie

(This is the full-strength chia smoothie on page 35 that I drink with 2 scoops of chia instead of one, but without the honey as I don't need the extra sweetness anymore.)

TOTAL CL: 17
TOTAL CALORIES: 314
INFLAMMATION: 832
ANDI: 3,228

2 scoops (1 ounce) chia:
Carb load 1
Calories 137
Inflammation 77
ANDI 68

½ cup nonfat Greek yogurt:
Carb load 4
Calories 60
Inflammation n/a
ANDI 30

½ cup blueberries:
Carb load 3
Calories 84
Inflammation –16
ANDI 130

3 cups raw kale:
Carb load 9
Calories 33
Inflammation 771
ANDI 1,000

Now compare the smoothie scores to those of a typical fast-food meal. In this meal there are more calories and a higher carb load than you'd want for a whole day. The meal is also highly inflammatory and bereft of nutrients, as you can see in the incredibly low ANDI score. Kale gives you an ANDI score of 1,000 with 33 calories, while this "All-American" meal scores you a pathetic 19 with more than 1,600 calories. You'll be left starving for micronutrients while your waistline swells.

The All-American

TOTAL CL: 72
TOTAL CALORIES: 1,623
INFLAMMATION: −116
ANDI: 19

1 large fast-food cheeseburger:
> Carb load 25
> Calories 800
> Inflammation n/a
> ANDI 11

1 large fries:
> Carb load 32
> Calories 495
> Inflammation n/a
> ANDI 7

1 large cola:
> Carb load 15
> Calories 328
> Inflammation −116
> ANDI 1

Here's a meal one might think is healthy, especially compared to fast food. However, look at the damage it does. The calories are nearly triple those in the chia smoothie. The inflammation is more than you should have in a week, and the nutrient content is nil, with an ANDI score of 208. A single serving of chard would hit 1,000. The French dressing loads you up with omega-6 fats, and the rice alone jacks up your CL by 24!

So-Called Healthy

TOTAL CL: 57
TOTAL CALORIES: 839
INFLAMMATION: −363
ANDI: 208

3 ounces cooked chicken breast tenders:

> Carb load 9
>
> Calories 210
>
> Inflammation −30
>
> ANDI 27

1 cup creamed corn:

> Carb load 18
>
> Calories 184
>
> Inflammation −107
>
> ANDI 44

1 cup white rice:

> Carb load 24
>
> Calories 242
>
> Inflammation −187
>
> ANDI 12

Small side salad:

1 cup iceberg lettuce:

> Carb load 1
>
> Calories 10
>
> Inflammation 7
>
> ANDI 110

¼ cup croutons:

> Carb load 4
>
> Calories 47
>
> Inflammation −22
>
> ANDI 15

2 tablespoons French dressing:

> Carb load 1
>
> Calories 146
>
> Inflammation −24
>
> ANDI n/a

Here's a truly healthy meal with reasonable calories and carb load and terrific anti-inflammatory qualities. However, even this meal can't beat the smoothie. The meal has a higher carb load and more calories.

Healthy

TOTAL CL: 27
TOTAL CALORIES: 485
INFLAMMATION: 517
ANDI: 1,190

1 cup cooked beans:
Carb load 14
Calories 227
Inflammation −45
ANDI 82

3 ounces cooked turkey breast:
Carb load 0
Calories 117
Inflammation −3
ANDI 25

½ cup mashed sweet potato:
Carb load 9
Calories 92
Inflammation 186
ANDI 83

1 cup cooked collards:
Carb load 4
Calories 49
Inflammation 379
ANDI 1,000

ROAD MAP:
TWO WEEKS OF AZTEC MEALS

The following recipes adhere to all the principles of the Aztec Diet so that the overall CL, inflammation, and omega-3 levels are right in the target zone. You may see a food that looks like it doesn't fit, but the overall plan allows it to work. The menus are just a guideline; pick and choose meals as you like. All the recipes you'll need for these meals are included in this chapter.

DAY 1

BREAKFAST

Spinach Basil Egg White Omelet

LUNCH

Salmon Salad on Sprouted Wheat Bread
Quinoa Tabbouleh

DINNER

Vegetable Red Lentil Soup with Kale and Collards

DAY 2

BREAKFAST

Quinoa Hot Cereal with Homemade Almond Milk and Blueberries

LUNCH

Curried Chicken Salad on a Sprouted Wrap
Arugula Salad with Apple Cider Vinaigrette

DINNER

Roasted Halibut with Parsley and Capers
Asparagus Ribbon Salad

DAY 3

BREAKFAST

Kale Egg White Frittata with Feta and Tomatoes

LUNCH

Asian Chicken Salad over Mixed Greens
Corn Soup

DINNER

Citrus Halibut over Roasted Kale

DAY 4

BREAKFAST

No-Dairy Vegetable Egg White Frittata

LUNCH

Mushroom Black Bean Soup with Kale
Mixed Green Salad with Dijon Vinaigrette

DINNER

Turkey Burgers
Roasted Broccoli

DAY 5

BREAKFAST

Mostly Egg White Frittata with Spinach and Goat Cheese

LUNCH

Walnut Red Pepper Spread on a Nori Wrap with Avocado
Spinach Salad, Pears, Walnuts, and Strawberry Balsamic Vinaigrette

DINNER

Roasted Curried Salmon
Mashed Celery Root

DAY 6

BREAKFAST

Salmon and Kale Frittata

LUNCH

Lentil Vegetable Soup with Spinach over Red Quinoa

DINNER

Lemon Pine Nut Crusted Salmon
Quinoa and Black Bean Salad with Cilantro Dressing

DAY 7

BREAKFAST

Vegetables and White Beans in Parchment with a Poached Egg on Top

LUNCH

White Beans and Tuna Salad over Bitter Greens with Creamy Coriander Vinaigrette
Simple Carrot Ginger Soup

DINNER

One-Pot Salmon with Kale and Quinoa

DAY 8

BREAKFAST

Vegetable Frittata Muffins

LUNCH

White Bean Hummus Open-Faced Sandwich
Massaged Kale Salad

DINNER

Salmon in Parchment
Brown Rice
Gingered Bok Choy

DAY 9

BREAKFAST
Chia Muesli

LUNCH
Herbed Poached Salmon Wrap with Low-Fat Tzatziki Sauce
Shaved Zucchini Salad

DINNER
Lemon Roasted Chicken with Seasonal Vegetables

DAY 10

BREAKFAST
Spiced Breakfast Amaranth with Homemade Almond Milk

LUNCH
Red Lentil Hummus on a Sprouted Tortilla with Avocado and Tomato
Summer Quinoa Salad with Lemon Cumin Vinaigrette

DINNER
Baked Quinoa and Walnut-Crusted Salmon
Kale Salad with Creamy Basil Avocado Dressing

DAY 11

BREAKFAST
Breakfast Crunch

LUNCH
Red Quinoa and Kale Cakes with Curried Yogurt Sauce
Spring Pea Salad

DINNER
Wood-Plank Cooked Salmon
Quick Braised Chard

DAY 12

BREAKFAST
High-Protein Flourless Almond Muffins

LUNCH
Black Bean Vegetable Stew over Red Quinoa
Spinach Salad with Strawberry Balsamic Vinaigrette

DINNER
Halibut with Peppers and Olives
Supersimple Collard Greens

DAY 13

BREAKFAST
Breakfast Burritos

LUNCH
Citrus Halibut or Salmon over Curried Millet Salad

DINNER
Turkey Meat Loaf
Roasted Cauliflower

DAY 14

BREAKFAST
Green Scrambled Egg Whites

LUNCH
Collard Wraps with Black Bean Salad
Quick Broccoli Leek Soup

DINNER
Nori-Wrapped Salmon
Herbed Quinoa
Sesame Asparagus

DAY 15

BREAKFAST

Breakfast Egg Drop Soup

LUNCH

Quick Lentil Vegetable Soup

Arugula and Spinach Salad with Strawberry Balsamic Vinaigrette

DINNER

Asparagus and Salmon Nori Wraps

ADDITIONAL CHOICES FOR BREAKFAST

Restorative Miso Soup

Salmon Cakes

Basic Vegetable Frittata—Build Your Own

RECIPES

These spectacular and imaginative recipes were created by Charlotte Hardwick, a truly inspiring chef. They make healthy meals that your whole family will love. We have not included scores for these recipes because they're comprised of the nutritious Premium Foods from the preceeding tables. Once you're choosing foods like these, you won't need to worry about numbers. Just enjoy.

Spinach Basil Egg White Omelet

4 egg whites

2 tablespoons nonfat milk

1 teaspoon chopped fresh basil

Pinch of sea salt

Pinch of freshly ground black pepper

1 teaspoon extra-virgin olive oil

1 teaspoon chopped scallion

¾ cup chopped fresh baby spinach

1 tablespoon grated Parmesan or crumbled goat cheese

1 teaspoon chopped fresh parsley

Combine the egg whites, milk, basil, salt, and pepper in a small bowl. Heat the olive oil in a skillet over medium heat, add the scallions, and cook, stirring, until softened. Add the spinach and stir to combine. When the spinach has wilted, pour the egg white mixture over the spinach. Lower the heat a little and watch as the edges begin to brown. When the edges are completely set, lift them gently with a spatula and tilt the skillet to allow the remaining egg mixture to run underneath and cook. Sprinkle the cheese on top and use the spatula to fold the omelet in half. Gently glide out of the pan and sprinkle with fresh parsley for garnish. Serve immediately.

SERVES 2

Salmon Salad

One 7-ounce can wild salmon
½ cup diced celery
½ small red onion, diced
2 tablespoons chopped fresh dill
1 tablespoon snipped fresh chives
3 tablespoons drained capers
2 tablespoons fresh lemon juice
2 tablespoons extra-virgin olive oil or plain nonfat Greek yogurt
Pinch of sea salt
Pinch of freshly ground black pepper

In a small bowl, combine the salmon, celery, onion, dill, chives, and capers. Whisk together the lemon juice, oil, salt, and pepper in another small bowl. Drizzle the vinaigrette over the salmon and toss gently to combine. Serve on sprouted wheat bread, over greens, or in a wrap.

SERVES 2

Quinoa Tabbouleh

2 cups water

1 cup quinoa

Sea salt

1 cucumber

1 tomato

1 bunch fresh mint

½ bunch fresh parsley

2 tablespoons fresh lemon juice

3 tablespoons extra-virgin olive oil

2 tablespoons snipped fresh chives

1 tablespoon pine nuts

1 tablespoon chia seeds

2 tablespoons crumbled feta cheese

Bring the water to a boil in a small saucepan. Rinse the quinoa and add to the boiling water with a pinch of sea salt. Reduce the heat and simmer, covered, for 20 minutes or until all the water is absorbed. Let the quinoa cool while you dice the cucumber and tomato. Chop the mint and parsley. Combine the quinoa with the vegetables and herbs. Mix gently and season with lemon juice, olive oil, and sea salt to taste. Sprinkle with the chives, pine nuts, chia seeds, and feta before serving.

This is delicious as a side salad, over mixed greens with a piece of fish, or in a wrap with lettuce for a portable lunch. Leftovers will keep in refrigerator for 2 to 3 days.

SERVES 4 TO 6

Vegetable Red Lentil Soup with Kale and Collards

2 tablespoons extra-virgin olive oil

1 medium onion

2 cups cubed, peeled sweet potato

2 teaspoons ground cumin

2 teaspoons ground coriander

2 teaspoons ground cinnamon

6 cups vegetable broth

2 cups dried lentils

One 14-ounce can fire-roasted tomatoes

Sea salt and freshly ground black pepper

1 cup kale ribbons (see Note)

1 cup collard ribbons (see Note)

Heat the olive oil in a soup pot over medium heat, and add the onion and spices. Cook for 5 minutes, until softened.

Stir in the broth, lentils, and tomatoes and season with salt and pepper to taste. Add kale, collards, and sweet potato, and cook for 5 more minutes or until the greens are wilted but still bright green. Reduce the heat to low and simmer until lentils and sweet potato are tender. Serve by itself as a soup or over red quinoa. It is delicious garnished with yogurt and slivered almonds.

Note: To make kale and collard ribbons, cut off the stems, stack the leaves, and roll the leaves up. Slice the rolls into thin ribbons.

SERVES 8 TO 10

Quinoa Hot Cereal

1 cup quinoa, rinsed

1½ cups water

1 cup almond milk, or more to taste

2 tablespoons chia seeds

Ground cinnamon

Handful blueberries (optional)

In a large saucepan, bring the quinoa, water, and almond milk (homemade, page 149, or store-bought) to a low boil; reduce to a simmer and cook until the water is absorbed, about 20 minutes. Stir in the chia. Put the cooked quinoa into a bowl and sprinkle with cinnamon to taste. Top with blueberries if desired and a little more almond milk if you want it a tad sweeter.

SERVES 3 TO 6; MAKES 3 CUPS COOKED QUINOA

Homemade Almond Milk

1 cup raw organic almonds
3 cups water, plus water for soaking
2 Medjool dates, pitted
1 teaspoon vanilla extract
Pinch of sea salt

Put the almonds in a big bowl and add enough water to cover. Let them sit overnight at room temperature. Drain and rinse. Add 3 cups fresh water to rinsed almonds in a blender and blend on high for 1 to 2 minutes. Add the pitted dates and vanilla and blend again. Pour the almond milk through a cheesecloth-lined colander into a wide-mouth pitcher or a bowl and then transfer to a pitcher. You may need a spatula to guide the milk through.

This will last for 3 to 4 days in the refrigerator and is a delicious substitute for cow's milk. You can double or triple this recipe easily to make as much as you need.

Variations

If you want a creamier almond milk, use 2 cups of water instead of 3. If you want it a little sweeter, add an extra pitted date or two.

MAKES 3 TO 4 CUPS

Curried Chicken Salad

4 boneless, skinless chicken breasts

2 tablespoons extra-virgin olive oil

Sea salt

7 tablespoons plain nonfat Greek yogurt

1 tablespoon fresh lemon juice

2 teaspoons curry powder

3 tablespoons snipped chives

¼ cup chopped fresh cilantro

Freshly ground black pepper

1 small Granny Smith apple, cored and cubed

2 tablespoons sliced almonds

Sliced scallions and chopped parsley for garnish (optional)

Preheat the oven to 375°F. Drizzle the chicken breasts with olive oil and sprinkle with sea salt. Roast in a shallow pan for 35 minutes. Whisk the yogurt, lemon juice, curry powder, chives, cilantro, 1 teaspoon salt, and pepper to taste to make a dressing. After the chicken is cooked and has cooled, shred or chop it and combine with the dressing. Fold in the apple and almonds. Serve over mixed greens and sprinkle with sliced scallions and fresh parsley if desired. This is also a good filling for a wrap when you need a portable lunch.

SERVES 4

Apple Cider Vinaigrette

3 tablespoons apple cider vinegar

2 teaspoons Dijon mustard

1 tablespoon minced shallot

¼ cup extra-virgin olive oil

Pinch of sea salt and freshly ground black pepper

Mix all ingredients to blend.

Roasted Halibut with Parsley and Capers

1 tablespoon chopped fresh parsley, plus parsley for garnish

1 tablespoon chopped fresh mint

1 tablespoon plain nonfat Greek yogurt

1 tablespoon drained capers

1 tablespoon grated lemon zest

Two 4- to 6-ounce skinless wild halibut fillets

Fresh lemon juice for serving

Preheat the oven to 350°F. Combine the herbs, yogurt, capers, and lemon zest in a small bowl and rub on the halibut. Bake in a shallow pan for 25 minutes and serve with or atop Asparagus Ribbon Salad. Top with parsley and a squeeze of lemon.

Variations

You can add chia seeds or sesame seeds to the yogurt-herb mixture to make a thicker crust.

SERVES 2

Asparagus Ribbon Salad

1 bunch fresh asparagus, tough ends snapped off

2 tablespoons fresh lemon juice

¼ cup extra-virgin olive oil

1 clove garlic, minced

Sea salt and freshly ground black pepper

With a vegetable peeler, start from the top of the asparagus spear and gently peel downward. Soon you'll have a pile of thin asparagus ribbons. When you get to the point where you have only a small bit of the asparagus, chop it into matchstick pieces. There is no wrong way to do this; you just want the asparagus to be thin because it's to be eaten raw.

Make a vinaigrette by whisking together the lemon juice, olive oil, and garlic. Drizzle over the asparagus and season with salt and pepper to taste. Let this sit for 30 minutes if you can.

Variations

To make this more of a meal than a side, place a mound of marinated asparagus on top of greens and sprinkle with walnuts, almonds, or sunflower seeds for crunch and protein. You can crumble a bit of feta on top or grate a bit of Parmesan over it or drizzle Lemon Tahini or Miso Tahini dressing (page 208) over it for a different flavor.

SERVES 2

Kale Egg White Frittata with Feta and Tomatoes

1 teaspoon extra-virgin olive oil, plus oil for the pan

½ cup chopped scallion

2 shallots, chopped

½ cup cherry tomatoes, halved or quartered

2 cups chopped stemmed kale

1 cup egg whites, whisked

2 tablespoons skim milk

Sea salt and freshly ground black pepper

¼ cup chopped fresh parsley

3 tablespoons crumbled feta cheese

Preheat the oven to 375°F. Lightly coat a 9-inch pie pan with olive oil. Heat the 1 teaspoon olive oil in a sauté pan or skillet over low heat, add the scallions and shallots, and cook until soft. Add the tomatoes and kale and cook until the kale is almost wilted. Turn off the heat and whisk together the egg whites, milk, and some salt and pepper. Add the kale mixture and stir. Add half of the parsley. Add the feta and pour the mixture into the prepared pie pan. Bake for 20 minutes or until golden brown. Cool and cut into wedges. Sprinkle with the remaining parsley and serve.

SERVES 3

Asian Chicken Salad

2 cups chopped roasted boneless, skinless chicken breast

1 cup chopped steamed and cooled asparagus or broccoli

½ cup diced red bell pepper

⅓ cup extra-virgin olive oil

¼ cup raw apple cider vinegar

1 teaspoon white sesame seeds

2 tablespoons honey

2 teaspoons tamari

½ cup chopped scallion

2 teaspoons chia seeds

2 teaspoons black sesame seeds

Combine the chicken and vegetables in a large bowl. Put olive oil, vinegar, white sesame seeds, honey, and tamari in a jar and shake to emulsify. Drizzle the dressing over the chopped chicken mixture and sprinkle with the scallions, chia seeds, and black sesame seeds. Serve over mixed greens.

SERVES 4

Corn Soup

2 tablespoons extra-virgin olive oil

2 cups frozen organic corn

1 small yellow onion, diced

½ cup sliced leek, white and light green parts only

Sea salt and freshly ground black pepper

3 cups vegetable stock or water

Chopped chives, parsley, or scallions for garnish (optional)

Heat the olive oil in a medium saucepan over medium heat. Add the corn, onion, and leeks and cook until softened. Season with sea salt and pepper to taste and stir. Add the stock and simmer for 30 minutes. Blend in batches in a blender or use an immersion blender to puree until smooth. Garnish with chives, parsley, or scallions.

SERVES 4

Citrus Halibut over Roasted Kale

Grated zest and juice of 1 lemon
Extra-virgin olive oil
Two 4- to 6-ounce skinless halibut fillets
1 bunch kale, leaves only
Sea salt

Preheat the oven to 375°F. Combine the lemon zest and juice with 1 tablespoon of olive oil and drizzle over the fish in a shallow pan. Tear the kale leaves into chip-sized pieces, put in a big bowl, and drizzle with enough olive oil to coat the leaves. Sprinkle with a pinch of salt and toss the leaves with your hands. Spread the kale on a large rimmed baking sheet. Roast the fish for 10 minutes, then add the kale to the oven. Roast the kale along with the fish for 5 minutes, then take the kale out of the oven and toss to cook the other side.

Return the pan to the oven for about 5 minutes and remove. Check the fish to make sure it is cooked through; if not, roast for up to another 5 minutes. Serve the fish on top of the kale.

SERVES 2

No-Dairy Vegetable Egg White Frittata

2 tablespoons extra-virgin olive oil, plus oil for the pan

2 tablespoons chopped scallion

¼ cup chopped broccoli

¼ cup chopped red bell pepper or tomato

6 egg whites, whisked

Pinch each of sea salt and freshly ground black pepper

Preheat the oven to 375°F. Lightly coat a 9-inch pie pan with olive oil. Warm the 2 tablespoons olive oil in a sauté pan or skillet over medium heat and add the scallion, broccoli, and red pepper and cook until softened. Transfer the vegetables to a bowl. Whisk or beat together the egg whites, salt, and pepper until foamy. Pour the egg whites over the vegetables and mix gently. Transfer to the prepared pan and bake for 15 minutes or until golden brown. Loosen the edges with a knife and cut into wedges before serving.

SERVES 4

Mushroom Black Bean Soup with Kale

2 tablespoons extra-virgin olive oil

1 large onion, diced

2 garlic cloves, minced

2 cups sliced mushrooms

2 pounds butternut squash or sweet potatoes, peeled and diced

1 cup drained and rinsed canned black beans

8 cups vegetable or chicken stock, or water

2 bay leaves

4 to 6 cups chopped and stemmed kale

Freshly ground black pepper and sea salt

Heat the olive oil in a sauté pan or skillet over medium heat and add the onion. Cook until soft. Add the garlic and cook for another minute or so. Add the mushrooms—you may have to work in batches, depending on how big your pan is. Add the squash and black beans and stir to combine. Next add the stock or water and bay leaves. Bring to a boil and skim the foam off the top. Reduce the heat and simmer for 30 to 60 minutes. If you are using water, it will make a nice vegetable stock the longer you let the vegetables simmer. Right before serving, stir in the kale and serve while the leaves are still bright green. Season to taste with pepper and salt.

You can use a variety of mushrooms in the soup. Shiitake and portobello mushrooms give the soup a rich flavor, but if you are pressed for time, you can buy sliced white and button mushrooms. This soup can be served as a side, main dish, or over quinoa as a hearty and immune-boosting meal.

SERVES 8

Dijon Vinaigrette

3 tablespoons champagne vinegar or apple cider vinegar

1 tablespoon minced shallot

½ teaspoon Dijon mustard

⅓ cup extra-virgin olive oil

Sea salt and freshly ground black pepper

Variations

Add ½ teaspoon chopped fresh thyme, mint, basil, or tarragon.

Turkey Burgers

1½ pounds lean ground turkey

¼ cup chia seeds

¼ cup orange juice

2 tablespoons fresh lime juice

3 tablespoons sesame seeds

¼ cup chopped scallion

3 tablespoons chopped fresh cilantro

2 tablespoons tamari

2 tablespoons chopped peeled fresh ginger

Sea salt and freshly ground black pepper to taste

Extra-virgin olive oil (optional)

Combine all the ingredients except the oil and form into 8 patties. Preheat the oven to 375°F or heat a little olive oil in a skillet. Bake or pan-cook the patties for 8 minutes on each side. Serve on a sprouted wheat bun or over greens.

MAKES 8 BURGERS

Roasted Broccoli

1 large head broccoli
2 tablespoons extra-virgin olive oil
Grated zest of 1 lemon
Sea salt

Preheat the oven to 400°F. Slice the head of broccoli and stem in half lengthwise down the center, then cut each half in half again. Repeat until you have relatively small slices of broccoli tops with long stems. Toss the broccoli with the oil, lemon zest, and salt to taste. Place on a baking sheet and roast for 20 minutes or until golden. This crispy broccoli is a huge hit with everyone!

SERVES 2

Mostly Egg White Frittata with Spinach and Goat Cheese

1 tablespoon extra-virgin olive oil
1 onion, chopped
2 cups fresh spinach
3 eggs
6 egg whites
1 ounce goat cheese, crumbled
1 tablespoon chopped fresh parsley

Preheat the oven to 375°F. In a 9- or 10-inch ovenproof skillet over medium heat, heat the oil, add the onion, and cook until softened. Add the spinach and cook until it wilts. Whisk the eggs and egg whites together and pour over the onion and spinach. Cook over low heat, running a spatula around the edges to prevent sticking and allow the uncooked eggs to run underneath and cook. Sprinkle with the cheese, transfer to the oven, and bake for 20 minutes or until golden brown. Loosen the edges with a spatula and slide onto a plate to cool. Cut into wedges and sprinkle with parsley before serving.

SERVES 6

Walnut Red Pepper Spread

½ cup walnuts

1 clove garlic

1 scallion, trimmed

½ cup plain nonfat Greek yogurt

½ cup chopped jarred roasted red peppers

1 tablespoon chia seeds

1 tablespoon chopped fresh basil

½ teaspoon hot red pepper flakes

Juice of 2 lemons

Sea salt and freshly ground black pepper to taste

Blend all ingredients in a blender or food processor until smooth and creamy. Spread on a sprouted tortilla with your favorite vegetables and wrap.

SERVES 2

Roasted Curried Salmon

One 4- to 6-ounce wild salmon fillet

2 teaspoons extra-virgin olive oil

1 teaspoon ground cumin

1 teaspoon curry powder

Sea salt

1 lemon

1 tablespoon chopped fresh cilantro

Preheat the oven to 350°F. Place the salmon on a baking sheet. Rub 1 teaspoon of the olive oil over the fish and sprinkle on the cumin, curry powder, and some salt. Cut lemon into 4 wedges and coat them with the remaining teaspoon of olive oil. Bake with the salmon for 20 to 25 minutes. Garnish with the cilantro and serve. You can also make a rub with olive oil, spices, and 1 tablespoon of chia seeds if you want a thicker crust on the fish.

SERVES 1 TO 2

Mashed Celery Root

Celery root (or celeriac) is a strange-looking root vegetable. Many people are intimidated by the way it looks, but it's a wonderful substitute for mashed potatoes.

> 2 pounds celery root, peeled and cubed
>
> Extra-virgin olive oil
>
> 1 cup vegetable stock
>
> Sea salt and freshly ground black pepper

Boil the celery root in water until tender. Drain and add back to the pot. Add enough stock to thin the mixture and olive oil to taste and beat with a beater as you would for mashed potatoes. Season with salt and pepper to taste and drizzle with a little olive oil before serving.

SERVES 8

Salmon and Kale Frittata

You can do all of this prep work the night before and keep the egg mixture covered in the refrigerator until you are ready to cook in the morning. You could easily substitute chopped asparagus for the kale if it is in season, or another green will work here too.

4 eggs

2 egg whites

Sea salt and freshly ground black pepper

Extra-virgin olive oil

½ cup diced scallion

2 cups chopped stemmed kale

2 teaspoons grated lemon zest, plus a little for garnish

2 teaspoons chopped fresh dill

Two 4-ounce cooked and cooled wild salmon fillets (see Note) or 4 ounces canned wild salmon

2 tablespoons crumbled low-fat feta cheese

Chopped fresh parsley for garnish

Beat the eggs and egg whites together in a large bowl. Season with salt and pepper. Heat the olive oil in a 9-inch ovenproof skillet over medium heat, add the scallions and kale, and cook until soft. Season with salt, pepper, lemon zest, and dill. Add the kale mixture to the eggs and stir.

Chop the cooled salmon into small pieces and add to the eggs. Add the feta and stir. Pour the egg mixture back into the pan and cook over medium-low heat until the edges start to set. Use your spatula to let the uncooked eggs run underneath and cook until set. Transfer to the oven and bake for 15 minutes or until golden brown. Garnish with fresh parsley and lemon zest. Cut and serve.

Note: Bake the salmon fillets at 350°F for 20 minutes.

SERVES 6

Lentil Vegetable Soup

2 cups dried lentils

3 tablespoons extra-virgin olive oil

2 cups chopped yellow onion

2 cups chopped leek, white parts only

1 cup diced celery

1 cup diced carrot

Sea salt and freshly ground black pepper

¼ cup tomato paste

6 cups water or vegetable stock

3 bay leaves

Rinse the lentils and put in a large pot with enough water to cover. Bring to a boil and skim foam off the top. Lower the heat and cook for 30 minutes, until soft.

In a large stockpot over medium heat, heat the oil and add the onion, leek, celery, and carrot until soft. Season with salt and pepper to taste and stir. Add the tomato paste and stir. Add the water or stock and bay leaves. Stir to combine, then add the cooked lentils. Bring to a boil and skim foam off the top. Reduce the heat and simmer, uncovered, for 30 minutes.

SERVES 4 TO 6

Herbed Red Quinoa

1½ cups red quinoa

3 cups water or vegetable stock

3 tablespoons extra-virgin olive oil

¼ cup chopped fresh parsley leaves

3 tablespoons chopped fresh thyme leaves

Sea salt and freshly ground black pepper

Rinse the quinoa well and drain. Transfer to a medium saucepan and add the water or stock. Bring to a boil and skim foam off the top. Reduce the heat to simmer, cover, and simmer until all the liquid is absorbed, 22 to 25 minutes. Season with the olive oil, herbs, and salt and pepper to taste. Stir and serve.

SERVES 4

Lemon Pine Nut Crusted Salmon

2 tablespoons Dijon mustard

Two 4- to 6-ounce skinless wild salmon fillets

Sea salt and freshly ground black pepper

¼ cup chopped pine nuts

2 tablespoons chopped fresh parsley

¼ cup chopped fresh basil

1 teaspoon chia seeds

Preheat the oven to 350°F. Spread the mustard on the salmon and season with salt and pepper. Combine the pine nuts, parsley, basil, and chia seeds and pat on top of the mustard-coated salmon. Bake for 20 to 25 minutes.

Variations

You can use almonds or walnuts instead of pine nuts if you prefer.

SERVES 2

Quinoa and Black Bean Salad

¾ cup quinoa

1½ cups water

Pinch of sea salt

3 cups cooked black beans

Cilantro Dressing (recipe follows)

1 cup cherry tomatoes, halved

Rinse and drain the quinoa. Bring the quinoa, water, and salt to a boil. Skim foam off the top, reduce the heat, cover, and simmer until all the water is absorbed, 15 to 20 minutes. Remove from the heat and set aside to cool. Place the black beans in a bowl with the cooled quinoa. Add the dressing and toss to combine. Fold in the tomatoes and stir.

SERVES 4 TO 6

Cilantro Dressing

3 tablespoons fresh lime juice

½ cup extra-virgin olive oil

1 garlic clove, minced

1 cup chopped fresh cilantro

Pinch of sea salt

½ teaspoon hot red pepper flakes

Put all the ingredients in a blender and pulse to combine.

Vegetables and White Beans in Parchment with a Poached Egg on Top

You can make packets the night before, then bake them in the oven as you poach your egg for an easy breakfast. You can also serve with scrambled egg whites if you prefer.

1 cup finely diced peeled sweet potato

½ cup diced yellow or orange bell pepper

½ cup diced red bell pepper

½ cup chopped spinach

¾ cup drained and rinsed canned white beans

1 teaspoon olive oil

1 teaspoon ground cumin

Pinch of freshly ground black pepper

Pinch of sea salt

Preheat the oven to 375°F. Lay two 15-inch squares of parchment paper or foil on a work surface. Combine the sweet potato, peppers, spinach, and beans in a medium bowl. Add the olive oil and cumin and toss to coat. Season with salt and pepper. Divide the vegetable mixture between the packets. Fold the paper or foil over the vegetables and seal the edges tightly to hold the vegetables inside. Transfer the packets to a rimmed baking sheet and bake for 25 to 30 minutes. Meanwhile, poach 2 eggs according to the directions that follow. Transfer the packets to plates and open them—be careful of steam—and add your poached egg on top. Enjoy this protein-and-fiber-rich breakfast.

Variation

You can use black beans in place of white beans.

SERVES 2

Perfect Poached Eggs

Always use the freshest eggs you can buy. Bring water in a saucepan almost to a boil. Add 2 teaspoons white or apple cider vinegar to the water. This will help the egg whites set. Then crack an egg into a small bowl and very gently drop the egg into the water. Use a spoon to gently guide the egg whites into the yolk. Turn off the heat and cover. Let the egg sit for about 3 minutes, depending on the size of the egg and how well done you want it to be. The egg whites should be cooked completely. Lift the egg out with a slotted spoon to drain and place on your vegetables.

Creamy Coriander Vinaigrette

¼ cup nonfat buttermilk

1 tablespoon champagne vinegar

3 tablespoons plain nonfat Greek yogurt

1 garlic clove, minced

1 teaspoon ground coriander

Mix all the ingredients to blend.

White Bean and Tuna Salad over Bitter Greens

One 15-ounce can organic white cannellini beans

One 6-ounce can light tuna packed in water

2 celery stalks, very thinly sliced

1 bunch radishes, tops removed, very thinly sliced

Creamy Coriander Vinaigrette (recipe follows)

1 small head radicchio

1 cup arugula

1 cup watercress or spinach

1 lemon

2 tablespoons extra-virgin olive oil

Freshly ground black pepper and sea salt

Chopped fresh parsley and chives for garnish

Drain and rinse the white beans and tuna. Put the beans, celery, and radishes into a bowl and drizzle with 2 tablespoons of the coriander dressing. Stir to combine. Break the drained tuna into big chunks and add to the white beans. Stir gently and add another tablespoon of dressing. Chop the radicchio and combine with the greens in a large bowl. Squeeze the lemon and drizzle the olive oil over greens. Season with salt and pepper to taste and toss. Top the greens with the tuna salad and garnish with parsley and chives.

Variations

You can also use canned wild salmon in this recipe if you prefer. Also feel free to substitute any of your other favorite greens. Use more of the coriander dressing instead of olive oil and lemon on the greens if desired.

SERVES 4

Simple Carrot Ginger Soup

3 tablespoons extra-virgin olive oil

1 yellow onion, chopped

3 tablespoons minced peeled fresh ginger

1 clove garlic, minced

Pinch of curry powder

Pinch of ground cinnamon

6 cups vegetable stock or water

1½ pounds carrots, peeled and chopped

Chopped fresh parsley for garnish

Heat the olive oil in a large pot over medium-low heat. Add the onion, ginger, and garlic and cook until softened. Add the curry and cinnamon and stir. Add the stock and the carrots. Heat to boiling. Skim foam off the top. Reduce the heat and simmer, uncovered, over medium heat until the carrots are very soft, about 30 minutes. Puree the soup with an immersion blender or in batches in a blender. Sprinkle with parsley before serving.

SERVES 6 TO 8

One-Pot Salmon with Kale and Quinoa

2 cups water

1 cup quinoa, rinsed

2 cups chopped stemmed kale

¼ cup chopped fresh mint

3 tablespoons chopped scallions

Grated zest and juice of 1 lemon

Sea salt and freshly ground black pepper

Four 4- to 6-ounce skinless wild salmon fillets

1 tablespoon extra-virgin olive oil

3 tablespoons walnuts

Preheat the oven to 425°F. In a 9 x 13-inch baking dish, mix together the water and the rinsed quinoa. Add the kale, mint, scallion, lemon zest, and sea salt.

Rub the salmon with the lemon juice and a small bit of olive oil. Season with salt and pepper. Place the salmon fillets on top of the quinoa mixture. Cover with foil and bake for 35 minutes, until the water has been absorbed and the fish is completely cooked through. Sprinkle the fish with walnuts before serving.

SERVES 4

Vegetable Frittata Muffins

Extra-virgin olive oil

12 egg whites

½ cup skim milk

Pinch of sea salt

Pinch of freshly ground black pepper

1 small onion, chopped

½ cup chopped mushrooms

½ cup chopped zucchini

¼ cup chopped red bell pepper

2 tablespoons chopped fresh basil

2 tablespoons chopped fresh parsley

2 tablespoons chia seeds

3 tablespoons grated Parmesan cheese

Preheat the oven to 350°F. Lightly oil 12 regular or 24 mini muffin cups or use paper liners. Whisk the egg whites, milk, salt, and pepper in a medium bowl until blended. Heat a little olive oil in a skillet or sauté pan over medium heat. Add the onion, mushrooms, zucchini, and red pepper and cook until soft. Add to the egg mixture. Add the basil, parsley, chia, and cheese. Spoon the mixture evenly into the prepared muffin cups. Bake for 20 minutes or until golden brown.

12 REGULAR OR 24 SMALL MUFFINS

White Bean Hummus Open-Faced Sandwich

2 cups cooked white beans

1 clove garlic

3 tablespoons extra-virgin olive oil

3 tablespoons tahini

3 tablespoons fresh lemon juice

Combine all the ingredients in a blender or food processor until smooth. If the hummus seems too thick, thin it with small amounts of water at a time until you get the consistency you want. It will thicken in the refrigerator.

Spread the hummus on a piece of sprouted wheat bread or millet bread and top with vegetables such as avocado slices, romaine leaves, chopped tomatoes, and grated carrots.

Variations

Sprinkle with a little ground cumin and minced fresh parsley before serving. Substitute black beans for white.

Massaged Kale Salad

1 small bunch kale
2 tablespoons extra-virgin olive oil
Sea salt
Fresh lemon juice

Stem the kale by pulling the leaves away from the stem. Stack the leaves on top of each other, roll up like a cigar, and cut into thin ribbonlike strips. Place the kale ribbons in a bowl and add olive oil and sea salt to taste. Massage the kale with the salt and olive oil until it wilts. This will break down the fibers and make it more digestible. Sprinkle with lemon to taste. This is a fun project for children, and they love this salad.

Variations

Add the Lemon Tahini Dressing on page 208 instead of olive oil and salt to massage into the kale and add toasted sunflower seeds, chia seeds, avocado, and apple.

SERVES 4

Salmon in Parchment

This is a great way to cook a fish that will easily fall apart on the grill. Cooking in parchment brings out flavors while preserving vitamins and minerals. It also makes little to no mess and will not make your house smell like fish!

One 4- to 6-ounce wild salmon fillet
Extra-virgin olive oil
Sea salt and freshly ground black pepper
Ground cumin
Ground ginger or minced peeled fresh ginger
Sliced lemon or orange
Sliced green or black olives

Preheat the oven to 375°F. Lightly rub the salmon with olive oil and season with salt, pepper, cumin, and ginger to taste. Cut a piece of parchment paper (12 x 16 inches) and lay on a clean work surface. Fold the paper in half, making a crease in the middle. Open and lay flat, placing the salmon at the center. Place lemon or orange slices over the salmon. Drizzle with olive oil and sprinkle with olives. Starting at a corner, fold the packet into a half moon and seal by joining the ends and folding them together. Transfer the packet to a baking sheet and cook for 20 to 25 minutes. You can add diced vegetables into the packets to cook with the fish. Just make sure they are small enough that they will cook completely.

Variations

You can cook as many packets as you like to make more servings.

SERVES 1

Brown Rice

1 cup short-grain brown rice

3 cups water

Pinch of sea salt

Rinse the rice in a strainer. Add the rice, water, and salt to a saucepan and bring to a boil. Skim the foam off the top. Reduce the heat to low, cover, and cook for 45 minutes, until all the water has been absorbed.

SERVES 3 TO 4

Gingered Bok Choy

1 tablespoon extra-virgin olive oil

½ onion, chopped

1 clove garlic, chopped

1 tablespoon chopped peeled fresh ginger

3 bunches bok choy, chopped

3 tablespoons water or vegetable broth

1 tablespoon fresh lemon or orange juice

1 tablespoon black sesame seeds

1 tablespoon chopped scallion, green part only

Heat the oil in a sauté pan or skillet, over medium heat, add the onion, and cook until soft. Add the garlic and ginger and stir. Add the bok choy and coat with onion and garlic mixture. Add the water and juice. Cook for 3 minutes, until the bok choy softens. Turn off the heat and add the sesame seeds and scallions to serve.

SERVES 2

Chia Muesli

2 tablespoons raw organic sesame seeds

2 tablespoons raw organic walnuts

2 tablespoons chia seeds

2 tablespoons raw organic almonds

¼ cup raw organic rolled oats

2 cups plain nonfat Greek yogurt

Ground cinnamon and fresh berries for garnish

Toss together the dry ingredients in a bowl. Pour the yogurt over the nut mixture and stir. Let the mixture sit in the refrigerator overnight. Scoop ½ cup of the mixture out for each serving and sprinkle with cinnamon and fresh berries to serve.

SERVES 4; MAKES 2 CUPS

Herbed Poached Salmon

This is an easy and healthy way to cook salmon and keep it very moist. It can be served over quinoa salad or greens, in a wrap, or over steamed greens for a low-fat dinner or lunch.

2 cups water
Sea salt and freshly ground black pepper
2 lemons, sliced
2 bay leaves
Two 4-ounce skinless wild salmon fillets
2 tablespoons chopped fresh flat-leaf parsley

Put the water in a large saucepan and season with some salt, one of the lemons, and the bay leaves. Bring to a low simmer and place the salmon in the liquid. Cook very gently for about 8 minutes. Remove the salmon from the water with a spatula and let all water drain off. Sprinkle with parsley and serve with the remaining lemon slices.

SERVES 2

Tzatziki Sauce

1½ cups plain nonfat Greek yogurt
1 English cucumber, peeled and seeded
1 tablespoon champagne vinegar
2 tablespoons fresh lemon juice
1 tablespoon extra-virgin olive oil
1 teaspoon minced garlic
2 teaspoons chopped fresh dill
Sea salt and freshly ground black pepper

Place the yogurt in a bowl. Dice the cucumber and add to the yogurt. Whisk in the vinegar, lemon juice, olive oil, garlic, dill, and salt and pepper to taste. This is really good after it sits overnight. Perfect for fish or chicken.

MAKES 2½ CUPS

Shaved Zucchini Salad

You can serve this as a main dish by adding salmon on top or add a little Parmesan cheese and more of your favorite vegetables to the salad.

1 zucchini

1 cup cherry tomatoes

¼ cup chopped raw walnuts or chopped raw almonds

2 tablespoons chopped fresh mint

2 tablespoons chopped fresh basil

Juice of 1 lemon

2 tablespoons extra-virgin olive oil

Sea salt and freshly ground black pepper

Trim the ends off the zucchini and use a vegetable peeler to peel the zucchini into thin ribbons. In a large bowl, combine the zucchini, tomatoes, walnuts, mint, and basil. Squeeze the lemon and drizzle the olive oil over the vegetables. Toss, season with salt and pepper to taste, and serve.

SERVES 2

Lemon Roasted Chicken with Seasonal Vegetables

One 4-pound organic chicken

2 tablespoons extra-virgin olive oil

Salt and freshly ground black pepper

1 small bunch fresh thyme, leaves only, chopped

Seasonal vegetables, such as sweet potato, squash, broccoli, cauliflower, and/or brussels sprouts

1 lemon, quartered

Preheat the oven to 375°F. Rinse and dry the chicken. Rub the chicken with 1 table-spoon of the olive oil, some salt and pepper, and the thyme. Roughly chop seasonal vegetables and place in a bowl. Toss with the remaining 1 tablespoon of olive oil. Place the chicken in a roasting pan or baking dish and spread the vegetables around the chicken. Insert lemon into cavity of chicken. Roast for 1½ hours, until the skin is golden brown, the juices run clear, and the meat is tender.

SERVES 4

Spiced Breakfast Amaranth

½ cup amaranth

1 cup almond milk

½ cup water

1 teaspoon vanilla extract

½ teaspoon ground ginger

½ teaspoon ground cinnamon

½ teaspoon ground nutmeg

Rinse and drain the amaranth. Spoon into a pot, add the almond milk and water, and bring to a boil. Skim the foam off the top and simmer, covered, over low heat for 20 to 25 minutes. Turn the heat off and let it sit for a minute to thicken. Add the vanilla and spices and stir. If you prefer a sweeter taste, add a sprinkle of stevia or a tablespoon of chopped goji berries.

SERVES 2

Red Lentil Hummus

1 cup dried red lentils

4 cups water

2 cinnamon sticks

2 tablespoons extra-virgin olive oil

1 small onion, chopped

¼ cup raw walnuts

1 teaspoon ground coriander

1 teaspoon ground cumin

1 teaspoon paprika

½ teaspoon cayenne

Sea salt

½ lemon

In a large pot, combine the lentils, water, and cinnamon sticks. Bring to a boil, skim foam off the top, reduce the heat to low, and cook, covered, for 30 minutes. Meanwhile heat the oil in a small sauté pan or skillet over medium heat, add the onion, and cook until soft. Add the walnuts, spices, and salt, and stir to combine. Drain the lentils into a bowl. Add the spiced onion mixture and stir. Puree in a blender or food processor or with an immersion blender. Finish with a squeeze of lemon. Spread on a sprouted wrap and fill with your favorite vegetables for a high-protein lunch on the go.

Red lentils cook very quickly, making this a fast, easy high-protein dip.

Summer Quinoa Salad with Asparagus and Lemon Cumin Vinaigrette

1 cup quinoa

2 cups water

2 tablespoons extra-virgin olive oil

¼ cup chopped scallion

1 cup chopped asparagus or zucchini

½ cup fresh or frozen corn

3 tablespoons chopped fresh basil

2 tablespoons chopped fresh parsley

Salt and freshly ground black pepper

Lemon Cumin Vinaigrette (recipe follows)

3 tablespoons chopped walnuts

Rinse and drain the quinoa. Place it in a saucepan with the water and bring to a boil. Reduce heat to low, cover, and simmer until all the water is absorbed, 15 to 20 minutes. Meanwhile, heat the oil in a small sauté pan or skillet over medium heat, add scallions and asparagus, and cook until soft. Add the corn and cook for 2 minutes. Turn off the heat and add the herbs and salt and pepper to taste. Stir. Combine the vegetables and quinoa. Add the vinaigrette and walnuts and stir.

SERVES 4

Baked Quinoa and Walnut-Crusted Halibut

Two 4- to 6-ounce skinless wild halibut fillets

2 teaspoons extra-virgin olive oil

Sea salt and freshly ground black pepper

1 cup cooked quinoa

3 tablespoons chopped walnuts

1 tablespoon chia seeds

2 tablespoons grated lemon zest

Preheat the oven to 350°F. Rub the halibut with 1 teaspoon of the olive oil and season with salt and pepper. Mix the quinoa, walnuts, chia seeds, the remaining teaspoon of olive oil, and the lemon zest together in a small bowl.

Place on top of the fish and bake for 20 to 25 minutes.

SERVES 2

Lemon Cumin Vinaigrette

2 tablespoons fresh lemon juice

⅓ cup extra-virgin olive oil

1 teaspoon ground cumin

Whisk together all the ingredients.

Kale Salad

8 ounces kale, stemmed and chopped

3 tablespoons Creamy Basil Avocado Dressing (recipe follows)

¼ cup toasted sunflower seeds

Put the kale leaves in a big bowl, drizzle the dressing over the greens, and toss to combine. Sprinkle the seeds over the top.

Variation

For a quick version of this salad, just squeeze lemon and 1 tablespoon of olive oil over the greens and toss. You can also add shredded carrots or radish over this for color and crunch.

SERVES 4

Creamy Basil Avocado Dressing

1 avocado

1 clove garlic, minced

2 tablespoons chopped fresh basil

2 tablespoons fresh lemon juice

2 tablespoons extra-virgin olive oil

Sea salt to taste

Water or champagne vinegar as needed

Spoon the flesh of one avocado into a blender and blend with the other ingredients. If the dressing seems too thick, thin with water or a little champagne vinegar.

Breakfast Crunch

¼ cup raw sunflower seeds

¼ cup raw sesame seeds

¼ cup raw pumpkin seeds

¼ cup chia seeds

1 cup raw walnuts

½ cup raw amaranth

1 cup raw quinoa

2 teaspoons ground cinnamon

1 teaspoon ground nutmeg

¼ cup extra-virgin olive oil

3 tablespoons maple syrup

Preheat the oven to 275°F. Pour all the dry ingredients onto a baking sheet and stir well. Mix the olive oil and maple syrup together and coat the mixture evenly. Spread into a thin layer. Bake for 20 minutes, take out and stir, and bake for 20 more minutes. Serve over nonfat yogurt and fresh berries.

MAKES 4 CUPS

Red Quinoa and Kale Cakes

1 cup red quinoa

2 cups water

4 eggs

1 teaspoon sea salt

1 teaspoon freshly ground black pepper

2 teaspoons ground cumin

2 teaspoons ground coriander

1 teaspoon paprika

1 cup chopped stemmed kale

½ cup chopped scallions

¼ cup chopped fresh dill or basil

2 tablespoons grated lemon zest

½ cup chia seeds

¼ cup crumbled goat cheese

Curried Yogurt Sauce (recipe follows)

Preheat the oven to 350°F. Rinse and drain the quinoa and add to a saucepan with the water. Bring to a boil. Skim the foam off the top, cover, and simmer until all the water is absorbed, 20 minutes (red quinoa takes a little longer to cook than white). While the quinoa is cooking, beat eggs with the salt, pepper, cumin, coriander, and paprika. Add the kale, scallions, dill, and lemon zest. Stir in the cooled quinoa and chia seeds. If the mixture needs more binding, add a little more chia or quinoa. Sprinkle in the goat cheese. Drop ¼-cup dollops of the mixture onto a baking sheet lined with parchment paper to form patties. Bake for 25 minutes, until brown. Serve with the yogurt sauce.

You can eat these cakes warm or freeze them once they've cooled to pull out for easy lunches and dinners. Serve over warm greens or atop salads.

MAKES 12 CAKES

Curried Yogurt Sauce

1 cup plain nonfat Greek yogurt

1 teaspoon ground cumin

1 teaspoon curry powder

1 tablespoon fresh lemon juice

Whisk all the ingredients together.

Spring Pea Salad

1 cup fresh or frozen edamame

Sea salt

1 cup fresh or frozen peas

1 cup fresh or frozen lima beans

1 tablespoon grated lemon zest

3 tablespoons fresh lemon juice

3 tablespoons champagne vinegar

¼ cup extra-virgin olive oil

2 scallions, finely chopped

3 tablespoons chopped fresh mint, plus more for garnish

2 tablespoons snipped fresh chives

Freshly ground black pepper

Cook the edamame in boiling salted water until crisp, about 4 minutes. Cook the peas in boiling salted water for 3 minutes and drain. Cook the lima beans in boiling salted water for 5 minutes and drain. Whisk together the lemon zest, lemon juice, vinegar, olive oil, scallions, mint, and chives. Pour the vinaigrette over the vegetables. Mix and season with salt and pepper to taste.

SERVES 4

Wood-Plank-Cooked Salmon

2 tablespoons extra-virgin olive oil

Two 4-ounce skinless wild salmon fillets

Juice of 1 lemon, plus more for serving

Sea salt

1 tablespoon chopped fresh parsley

Brush a wood plank with a tablespoon of the olive oil. Put the plank in the oven and preheat to 350°F for 15 to 20 minutes to warm the plank. Season the salmon with the remaining olive oil, the lemon juice, and some sea salt. Remove the warm plank from the oven, place the salmon on the plank, and bake for 25 minutes. Season with parsley and more lemon juice or serve with a dollop of low-fat Tzatziki Sauce (page 177).

Variation

You can also use this method to roast a whole salmon fillet and serve at the table on the plank.

SERVES 2

Quick Braised Chard

1 pound chard
1 tablespoon extra-virgin olive oil
1 garlic clove, thinly sliced
1 tablespoon water
Fresh lemon juice
Sea salt and freshly ground black pepper

Strip the chard leaves from the stalks and reserve the stalks for another use. Chop the greens. Heat the olive oil in a large skillet over medium heat, add the garlic, and cook until golden. Add greens. Stir to coat with the olive oil and add the water. Cook until the chard is wilted. Season with lemon, salt, and pepper to taste.

Variation
Substitute vinegar for lemon and onion for garlic.

SERVES 2

High-Protein Flourless Almond Muffins

1½ cups raw almonds or almond meal
¼ cup almond milk
¼ cup maple syrup
6 egg whites
1 teaspoon vanilla extract
1 teaspoon ground cinnamon
½ teaspoon sea salt
¼ cup chia seeds

Preheat the oven to 375°F and line muffin cups with paper liners. Grind the almonds in a food processor until they are finely ground like a flour or use store-bought almond meal. Whisk or beat together the almond milk, maple syrup, egg whites, vanilla, cinnamon, and salt. Add the ground almonds and chia. Stir until everything is combined. Pour the batter into paper-lined muffin cups. Bake for 20 minutes or until golden brown.

MAKES 12 REGULAR MUFFINS OR 18 SMALL MUFFINS

Black Bean Vegetable Stew

1 to 2 tablespoons extra-virgin olive oil

1 medium onion, chopped

1 teaspoon ground cinnamon

2 teaspoons ground cumin

1 teaspoon ground coriander

1 teaspoon cayenne

1 teaspoon chili powder

2 cups chunks of peeled butternut squash or sweet potato

1 cup frozen or fresh corn

4 cups vegetable stock or water

One 14-ounce can chopped tomatoes

2 cups rinsed and drained canned black beans

½ cup chopped jarred roasted red bell peppers

In a large stockpot over medium heat, heat the olive oil, add the onion, and cook until soft. Add all the spices, stir to mix, and add the squash, corn, stock, and tomatoes. Stir and simmer for 30 minutes. Add the black beans and red peppers and simmer for 5 more minutes. Serve over red quinoa.

SERVES 6 TO 8

Halibut with Peppers and Olives

Two 4-ounce skinless wild halibut fillets

Extra-virgin olive oil

Sea salt and freshly ground black pepper

½ small onion, chopped

½ cup chopped red bell pepper

½ cup chopped yellow bell pepper

1 teaspoon chopped fresh rosemary

1 teaspoon chopped fresh thyme leaves

¼ cup white wine or vegetable broth

½ cup chopped kalamata olives

2 tablespoons chopped fresh parsley

Preheat the oven to 350°F. Brush the halibut with olive oil and sprinkle with salt and pepper. Place on a baking sheet and roast for 25 minutes. While the fish is roasting, heat 1–2 tablespoons of olive oil in a sauté pan or skillet over medium heat, add the onion, peppers, rosemary, and thyme, and cook until soft. Add the wine and cook for 2 minutes. Stir in the chopped olives and parsley. Top the halibut with this delicious tapenade and serve.

SERVES 2

Supersimple Collard Greens

2 tablespoons extra-virgin olive oil

½ onion, chopped

1 clove garlic, chopped

1 pound collard greens

Water

1 tablespoon apple cider vinegar or fresh lemon juice

Heat 1 tablespoon of the olive oil in a large skillet over medium heat, add the onion, and cook until soft. Add the garlic and cook for another minute or two. Remove the collard leaves from the stems. Stack the leaves, roll up like a cigar, and cut into thin ribbons. Add the collards to the onion and enough water to cover. Put on lid. Cook for 3 minutes or until wilted but still bright green. Add the vinegar and the remaining tablespoon of olive oil and stir.

SERVES 2

Breakfast Burritos

1 tablespoon extra-virgin olive oil

1 small onion, chopped

1 scallion, chopped

½ green bell pepper, chopped

½ cup chopped tomato

½ cup sliced mushrooms

4 egg whites

1 teaspoon ground cumin

½ teaspoon ground coriander

¼ teaspoon cayenne

Pinch of sea salt

Pinch of freshly ground black pepper

¼ cup chopped fresh cilantro

Heat the olive oil in a sauté pan or skillet over medium heat. Add the onion and scallion and cook until soft. Add the green pepper, tomato, and mushrooms and cook until tender. Whisk in egg whites and cook until eggs are slightly scrambled. Add spices and salt and pepper. Spoon into sprouted or corn tortillas and garnish with cilantro. Roll up and enjoy!

SERVES 2 TO 4

Citrus Halibut or Salmon

Grated zest and juice of 1 lemon

1 tablespoon extra-virgin olive oil

Two 4- to 6-ounce skinless wild halibut or salmon fillets

1 scallion, green part only, chopped, for garnish

Chopped fresh parsley for garnish

Preheat the oven to 375°F. Combine the lemon zest and juice with the olive oil and drizzle over the fish. Bake for 20 to 25 minutes. Garnish with the scallion and parsley. For a beautiful lunch, serve the fish topped with roasted lemon slices.

SERVES 2

Curried Millet Salad

Millet is a gluten-free grain high in protein and iron.

1 cup millet

3 cups water

¼ cup plain nonfat Greek yogurt

¼ cup extra-virgin olive oil

3 tablespoons red wine vinegar

2 tablespoons curry powder

1 teaspoon sweet paprika

Pinch of sea salt

Freshly ground black pepper

1 cup chopped baby spinach

½ cup diced carrot

¼ cup chopped almonds

2 scallions, white parts only, chopped

¼ cup chopped fresh parsley

Rinse the millet, combine with the water in a saucepan, and bring to a boil, Reduce the heat to low and simmer for 30 minutes or until all the liquid is absorbed. While the millet is cooking, whisk together the yogurt, olive oil, vinegar, curry, paprika, salt, and pepper. Pour this mixture over the millet and mix well. Stir in the spinach, carrots, almonds, scallions, and parsley.

SERVES 4

Turkey Meat Loaf

1 to 2 tablespoons extra-virgin olive oil

1 onion, chopped

2 tablespoons tomato paste

2 tablespoons mustard

2 pounds ground organic turkey breast

3 large eggs, beaten

1½ cups cooled cooked quinoa

½ cup chia seeds

1 cup chopped spinach

1 cup chopped kale

Preheat the oven to 350°F. Heat the olive oil in a sauté pan or skillet over medium heat, add the onion, and cook until soft. Add the tomato paste and mustard to make a paste. Set aside to cool.

In a large bowl, combine the turkey, cooled onion mixture, eggs, cooled quinoa, chia seeds, and chopped greens. Put in a 9 x 5-inch loaf pan and bake for 45 to 60 minutes.

SERVES 8

Roasted Cauliflower

1 head cauliflower
Juice of ½ lemon
Extra-virgin olive oil
Sea salt and freshly ground black pepper

Preheat the oven to 400°F. Cut the cauliflower into florets and put on a parchment-lined baking sheet. Squeeze the lemon juice and drizzle with some olive oil over the cauliflower. Season with salt and pepper to taste and bake for 25 to 30 minutes or until golden brown.

Variations
You can add any spice or herb you like to the olive oil before drizzling. This is also delicious sprinkled with chia and/or sesame seeds after cooking.

SERVES 4

Green Scrambled Egg Whites

3 egg whites
1 teaspoon extra-virgin olive oil
½ cup chopped spinach
Sea salt and freshly ground black pepper
1 tablespoon chopped fresh parsley or scallion

Whisk or beat the egg whites in a clean bowl until soft peaks form. Heat the olive oil in a sauté pan or skillet over medium heat, add the spinach, and cook until it begins to wilt. Add the egg whites to the pan and cook over low to medium heat until the desired consistency. Season with salt and pepper. Garnish with parsley or scallions and serve over sprouted toast.

SERVES 1

Collard Wraps with Black Bean Salad

If jícama is hard to find, you can omit or replace with diced carrots or celery.

1 cup cooked black beans

½ cup chopped peeled jícama

½ cup corn kernels

¼ cup chopped fresh basil and/or cilantro

¼ cup chopped tomato

Juice of 1 lime

2 tablespoons extra-virgin olive oil

Sea salt and freshly ground black pepper to taste

Combine all the ingredients to make black bean salad.

To wrap in a collard leaf: Wash collards and remove the thick stems from the bottom of each leaf. In a large skillet, simmer 1 inch of water and put a collard leaf in the simmering water for about 5 seconds on each side. They will turn a beautiful bright green color. Take out with tongs and lay on a paper towel to dry.

You can repeat process and lay another collard on top for a thicker wrap or just use one to wrap your filling. Put your black bean filling in the middle of the collard and slice some avocado on top. Leave enough space around the edges so you can roll them up. Roll toward the center and roll tightly. You can then wrap in foil or parchment.

SERVES 2

Variation
If you want a quicker wrap option, try a corn tortilla with shredded cabbage and avocado.

Quick Broccoli Leek Soup

3 tablespoons extra-virgin olive oil

3 cups chopped leek, white part only

8 cups broccoli florets

4 to 5 cups water or vegetable stock

Sea salt and freshly ground black pepper

Plain nonfat Greek yogurt and grated lemon zest for garnish (optional)

Heat the olive oil in a large sauce pan over medium heat, add the leek, and cook until soft. Add the broccoli and stir to combine. Add the water. Bring to a boil and skim foam off the top. Lower the heat and simmer until the broccoli is cooked. Puree the soup, working in batches, in a blender or with an immersion blender in the pot. Season with salt and pepper. Serve with a little dollop of nonfat Greek yogurt and lemon zest on top.

Variation

This recipe is a basic technique for any pureed vegetable soup. You could also use butternut squash, carrot-ginger, cauliflower, or mushroom.

SERVES 4

Nori-Wrapped Salmon

1 tablespoon extra-virgin olive oil

Juice of ½ lemon

1 tablespoon finely chopped fresh dill

1 tablespoon chia seeds

Sea salt and freshly ground black pepper

Two 4- to 6-ounce skinless wild salmon fillets

2 sheets nori

Preheat the oven to 375°F. Mix the oil, lemon juice, dill, chia seeds, and some salt and pepper together and spread on the salmon. Lay the nori on the kitchen counter and place the salmon oiled side down in the middle of the nori sheet. Wrap the salmon with the nori until it is fully covered. It is almost like you are wrapping a present! Place the salmon on a baking sheet lined with parchment and bake for 20 to 25 minutes.

SERVES 2

Herbed Quinoa

1½ cups red quinoa

3 cups water or vegetable stock

3 tablespoons extra-virgin olive oil

¼ cup chopped fresh basil leaves

¼ cup chopped fresh parsley leaves

3 tablespoons chopped fresh thyme leaves

Sea salt and freshly ground black pepper

Rinse the quinoa well and drain. Place in a medium saucepan with the water. Bring to a boil and skim foam off the top. Reduce the heat to simmer, cover, and cook until all the liquid is absorbed, 12 to 15 minutes. Season with olive oil, herbs, and salt and pepper to taste. Stir before serving.

SERVES 4

Sesame Asparagus

1 bunch asparagus

¼ cup water

2 tablespoons tahini

3 tablespoons extra-virgin olive oil

1 tablespoon tamari

1 tablespoon fresh lemon juice

1 tablespoon plain nonfat Greek yogurt

1 teaspoon minced peeled fresh ginger

2 tablespoons black sesame seeds

Snap off the tough ends of the asparagus and discard. Bring the water to a boil in a saucepan and add the asparagus. Cover and cook for 2–3 minutes, until bright green and crisp. Drain. In a blender, combine remaining ingredients except the sesame seeds and blend until creamy. Coat the drained asparagus with the sauce and sprinkle with black sesame seeds.

SERVES 2 TO 3

Breakfast Egg Drop Soup

This soup is warm and nourishing, and even children love it! You can add an extra egg white for protein or more greens and less egg.

3 cups chicken or vegetable stock

3 eggs

1 egg white

2 scallions, finely chopped

½ cup baby spinach

Sea salt and freshly ground black pepper

Chopped fresh parsley for garnish

Heat the broth in a saucepan over medium heat. Whisk the eggs and egg white together in a glass measuring cup. Add the scallions (saving a few pieces for garnish) and spinach to the broth and stir. Let that mixture simmer for 5 minutes. Pour the eggs into the soup in a thin stream, whisking the soup as you pour. Season with salt and pepper. Pour into the bowls and garnish with a few scallions and the parsley.

SERVES 4

Quick Lentil Vegetable Soup

4 cups water or broth

1 cup dried lentils

1 sweet potato

2 carrots

2 stalks celery

1 onion

1–2 tablespoons extra-virgin olive oil

1 teaspoon ground cumin

1 teaspoon ground coriander

1 teaspoon mustard seeds

Combine the water and lentils in a saucepan. Bring to a boil, skim foam off the top, and simmer over low heat for 25 to 30 minutes. Meanwhile peel and dice the sweet potato, carrots, celery, and onion. Heat the oil in another saucepan over medium heat, add the diced vegetables, and cook until soft. Stir in the cumin, coriander, and mustard seeds. Add the cooked lentils and heat to serve.

SERVES 6 TO 8

Arugula and Spinach Salad with Strawberry Balsamic Vinaigrette

5 large ripe strawberries, stems removed, finely chopped

3 tablespoons balsamic vinegar

⅓ cup extra-virgin olive oil

Sea salt and freshly ground black pepper

Large handful of arugula

Large handful of spinach

Place strawberries in a small bowl with vinegar and let sit for 15 minutes. Whisk or blend in the oil and season with salt and pepper. Place the greens in a bowl and drizzle with the dressing. You will have dressing to spare. Leftovers will keep for a few days.

Asparagus and Salmon Nori Wraps

1 pound asparagus spears, tough ends snapped off, diced

4 ounces smoked wild salmon or 1 roasted 4-ounce piece wild salmon

6 nori wrappers

1 ripe avocado, sliced

¼ cup shredded carrot

¼ cup shredded cabbage

1 teaspoon chia seeds

¼ cup chopped fresh basil

¼ cup chopped fresh mint

Cover the bottom of a skillet with water and bring to a boil. Add the asparagus, cover, and cook until tender, about 2 minutes. Drain and set aside. Cut the salmon slices into thin strips or crumble the roasted salmon into the center of each nori wrapper. Sprinkle asparagus into the center on top of the salmon. Add the rest of the vegetables then chia, and the herbs. Drizzle with a vinaigrette or lemon juice and wrap the nori tightly in a cone shape. Seal the edges with a little water. Serve fresh or wrap in parchment for lunch on the go.

SERVES 2 OR 3; MAKES 6 WRAPS

Restorative Miso Soup

3 cups water or vegetable stock

3 kale leaves, stemmed and chopped

⅛ cup organic white miso

2 scallions, chopped

1 sheet nori

Hot red pepper flakes for garnish (optional)

Chopped fresh cilantro for garnish (optional)

Bring the water to a boil. Add the kale and simmer for 10 to 15 minutes, until bright green and tender. Remove from the heat. In a small bowl, dissolve the miso in enough water to thin it out and make a paste. The amount of water will depend on the texture of the miso. Pour the kale soup into bowls. Spoon 2 tablespoons of dissolved miso into each soup bowl. Crumble the nori over the soup bowls. Garnish with red pepper flakes and/or cilantro if you like.

Variations

You can replace the kale with any green. Watercress and bok choy are perfect for a cleansing soup. Baby spinach works well when you are pushed for time. You can add fish or egg whites for extra protein.

SERVES 2 TO 4

Salmon Cakes

These freeze really well if you want to double the batch and save some for an easy breakfast or lunch.

One 7.5-ounce can wild salmon

⅛ cup chia seeds

2 tablespoons sesame seeds

Juice of ½ lemon

3 tablespoons plain nonfat Greek yogurt

1 tablespoon chopped fresh dill

1 tablespoon extra-virgin olive oil

Drain and rinse the salmon. Be sure to remove any skin or tiny bones. In a bowl, add all the other ingredients except the oil to the salmon and mix. Form the mixture into 4 equal patties. Heat the olive oil in a skillet over medium heat and add the salmon cakes. Cook for 3 to 4 minutes on each side or until golden brown. Serve alone with a squeeze of lemon and a sprinkle of dill or alongside scrambled egg whites.

MAKES 4 CAKES

Basic Vegetable Frittata—Build Your Own

If you like to play around in the kitchen, here is a blueprint for a frittata to which you can add any seasonal vegetable, any cheese, and any herb you like.

    2 tablespoons extra-virgin olive oil
    ½ cup chopped scallion, leek, or onion or 1 tablespoon chopped shallot or garlic
    1¼ cup chopped vegetables
    4 eggs
    2 egg whites
    ¼ cup skim milk
    3 tablespoons grated or crumbled cheese
    Sea salt and freshly ground black pepper
    ¼ cup chopped herb or a combination of herbs
    Chopped scallions and fresh parsley for garnish

Preheat the oven to 350°F. In a large ovenproof sauté pan or skillet (9- or 10-inch), heat the olive oil over medium heat. Add the scallion and cook until soft. Add the vegetables and cook until they begin to brown. Whisk the eggs and egg whites in a large bowl with the milk, cheese, and some salt and pepper. Stir in the vegetables and herbs and pour back into the pan. Cook until the edges begin to set and then run a spatula around the edges to let some of the egg run underneath and cook a little. Transfer the pan to the oven and cook for 10 to 15 more minutes or until golden brown. Let cool and slice into wedges. Garnish with scallions and parsley.

Vegetables that work well in frittatas include zucchini, cauliflower, squash, peppers, mushrooms, onions, broccoli, spinach, kale, and chard. For herbs, try parsley, basil, dill, marjoram, and cilantro. For cheeses, experiment with Parmesan, feta, and goat.

SERVES 6 TO 8

ADDITIONAL DRESSINGS

All of these dressings can be whisked together in a bowl, poured into a jar and shaken, or blended in a blender. Mix the vinegar or juice with the seasonings first, then add the oil and mix to emulsify. Add any sea salt and pepper at the end, to taste.

Sesame Vinaigrette

1 tablespoon minced peeled fresh ginger

1 tablespoon minced shallot

3 tablespoons rice vinegar

2 teaspoons tamari

¼ cup grapeseed oil

1 tablespoon sesame seeds

Lemon Tahini Dressing

⅓ cup tahini

3 tablespoons fresh lemon juice

¼ cup water

1 tablespoon extra-virgin olive oil

1 teaspoon grated lemon zest

Miso Tahini Dressing

Miso is a probiotic and flushes away toxins. This is a great dressing to drizzle over steamed vegetables and will replenish and build healthy intestinal flora.

1 shallot, minced

1 clove garlic, minced

3 tablespoons fresh lemon juice

2 tablespoons miso

½ cup extra-virgin olive oil

CHAPTER 10

LIFE ON PHASE III

AD ALUMNI

Fueling yourself with the clean, energizing foods you've learned about in Phase Three radically transforms your life. Shedding excess weight, dumping carb bombs, and dousing the fires of inflammation gives you a totally new look and a totally new outlook. You may not even have realized how bad you felt until you started feeling better. Now that sluggish feeling is gone. You are no longer at the mercy of cravings for overly sweet, salty, artificially flavored, processed foods. Your body, your mood, your health, and your whole life improve as a result.

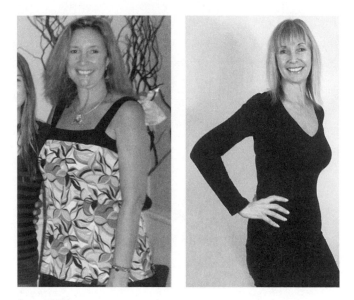

Susan Szabo
65, Kailua, Oahu
Beginning weight: 174 pounds
End weight: 130 pounds
Weight lost: 44 pounds

"I eat less because I crave less sugar. It's absolutely phenomenal. Walking on the beach used to feel hard, now it feels easy . . . I'm happy, optimistic!"

Susan Szabo, an artist in Kailua, Oahu, likened the change in her body to trading a big dirty bus for a clean, new little Mini Cooper. "I feel light. I can see through the windshield. I'm happy, optimistic. I've never felt that before!" she said. Susan recently went to the airport and lugged her suitcase onto the scale at check-in. It weighed 42 pounds. "That is what I'd been carrying around," she said. Soon to be sixty-five, Susan said she feels healthier than ever in her life.

Chia smoothies helped Susan stop craving sugar and therefore eat less, she said. But she discovered other significant benefits as well. In 2009 carpel tunnel syndrome had kept Susan from painting, which is her passion and her livelihood, for six months. She also suffered from low-grade chronic depression and had spent nine years on various antidepressants. Ten days after Susan started adding chia to her breakfast smoothie, her carpel tunnel syndrome disappeared. Inflammation, gone! She was also thrilled when she learned about the high levels of omega-3s in chia and their successful use in treating depression. By early 2012, Susan had been off antidepressants and depression-free for two years. She had also lost 44 pounds. "It was absolutely phenomenal," she said.

Great things happen when junky foods stop ruling your world. You feel thin, happy, energetic, calm, and confident. Phase Three of the Aztec Diet is simple and straightforward, not a diet at all but a way of life. You are eating real, whole foods that have sustained centuries of smart, energetic, successful people. You don't have to count calories or points or order expensive, special foods. Now and then you can indulge in something totally decadent and unhealthy because your regular eating habits are so good that it won't make a bit of difference.

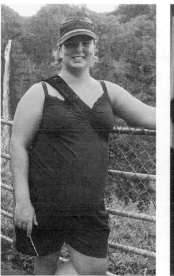 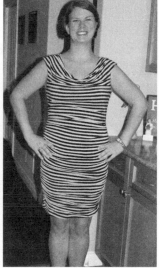

Corie van Biert
31, Nanaimo, BC, Canada
Beginning weight: 252 pounds
Current weight: 174 pounds (and still going!)
Weight loss: 78 pounds

FREQUENTLY ASKED QUESTIONS

Do I still drink chia smoothies?

Sure! Smoothies make a great meal or snack whether you're dieting or not, because they're quick, easy, and nutritious. Have one every day for breakfast or just once in a while. It's up to you. I do recommend returning to Phase Two of the AD when you need to recover from indulging yourself on a vacation or holiday. A couple of days on Phase Two (Phase One if you really overdid it) will bring you right back to where you belong. If you need a quick recovery from a big dinner out, make a chia smoothie for breakfast.

You can also drink chia in water or a sports drink before or during your workout. Sprinkle it on cereal or yogurt or add it to your favorite recipes. Don't leave it behind in Phase Three. It really is a supergrain.

Do I need to count calories or carb load?

No. Of course you don't want to eat too many calories or pump your carb load sky-high, or you'll be right back where you started. Get to know the premium food tables in Chapter 8 so you're aware of the carb loads of common foods. Pay special attention to the Substitution Chart. If you're eating primarily the premium foods in this book, you shouldn't need to count at all.

I still sometimes crave pancakes (or cheeseburgers or ice cream or pizza). What should I do?

Eat them! Satisfy your craving and leave it behind you. This is the beauty of the Aztec Diet. Your regular eating habits are now so good that splurging here and there won't hurt you. If you gain a few pounds, go back to Phase One or Two until they're gone. Just be careful not to go on such a food bender that you get caught back in the cycle of peaking and plunging blood sugar.

What about alcohol?

Cut out alcohol while you're dieting, but once you've reached your target weight, feel free to enjoy alcohol in moderation. Don't drink late into the night as alcohol will mess with your metabolism and your sleep. Drink early and judiciously. Red wine has a carb load of zero!

I have children, and dinner is an important part of our family life. How can I incorporate the Aztec Diet into our routine?

Choose premium foods from Chapter 8 or try some meals from Chapter 9 and eat dinner early. If your children need to adjust gradually to healthier fare, consult the Substitution Chart in Chapter 8 so you can keep yourself on track when you're cooking Western foods for others. Just substituting Aztec grains for carb bombs and incorporating some high-scoring veggies will improve your health and your family's health enormously.

CHAPTER 11

THE BIG PICTURE

The Aztec Diet has given you a lean physique and calm, steady energy. Now it's time to look at the bigger picture. The benefits you've reaped from the AD can be enhanced by two other factors that impact your health and well-being enormously: sleep and exercise. Together the right diet, sleep habits, and exercise routine can improve every aspect of your life. Your mood, productivity, relationships, and health will flourish, allowing you to make the most of every day of your life.

SLEEP MATTERS

A good night's sleep is key to weight management—in fact, lack of sleep is closely linked to obesity in research studies[1]—but millions of Americans have trouble sleeping. Sleep experts say that most problems stem not from disorder or disease but from poor sleep hygiene. This section will help you achieve good sleep hygiene, which simply means having control over all the factors, behavioral and environmental, that can wreck a good night's sleep. We don't sleep in solid blocks of eight or so hours, but drift in cycles between states of deep sleep and arousal. (If you've ever trained a baby to sleep through the night, you know all about this!) Having a good night's sleep means that the cycles of deep sleep are as long and sound as possible. The following tips will help you get the most restorative sleep so you'll wake up well rested and alert.

Exercise is the first precursor to healthy sleep. A late-afternoon or early-evening workout is a great way to set up your night. Late-night exercise may keep you up. However, practicing yoga before bed helps your mind and body wind down. If I watch TV at night, I go through all the Bikram yoga poses while I watch.

Banish stimulants close to bedtime. (Close can mean 12 hours away!) Stimulants will doom your sleep. I drink my last caffeine at 11:00 A.M. If you smoke, try to have your last cigarette in the early afternoon—or, better yet, quit!

Alcohol does speed the onset of sleep but badly disrupts sleep in the second half of your night as your body metabolizes it. If you're not sleeping well, give up alcohol until you've mastered a good night's sleep; then drink judiciously and early.

Certain foods may keep you up, such as spicy foods; chocolate, which has hidden caffeine; and milk or ice cream if you're lactose intolerant. Be wary of these at dinner and don't eat them late at night.

Too much food for dinner will destroy the architecture of deep sleep, waking you often during the night. Eat no more than 250 calories after 6:00 P.M. and go to bed hungry. You'll get a terrific night's sleep and wake up hungry, ready for a healthy, energizing chia smoothie.

Night eating syndrome is more than just too much food for dinner; it's a real disease that has been widely researched lately. If you eat more than 50 percent of your daily calories after 6:00 P.M., you've got it. Many people who struggle with their weight suffer from night eating syndrome. These are the symptoms:

- No morning hunger

- Reduced daytime hunger

- Trouble sleeping

- Stressful days

- Carb cravings in the evening

- Disproportionate number of calories eaten at night

Night eating syndrome can cause low self-esteem and even depression. For others it totally derails a day of very healthy eating, making weight control impossible. Conquering night eating syndrome is the number one thing that can help you break the cycle of obesity. It won't happen right away. The more you can project forward and think about an amazing morning as your ultimate reward, the better you'll get at managing your evening appetite. If you nap during the day and have trouble sleeping at night, stop. Make sure you're tired enough to go to sleep and turn in early so you don't have to resist the lure of the refrigerator.

Turn off electronic stimuli two hours before bed. Many of us force ourselves to stay up hours later than we should with the help of electronic stimuli. Texting, tweeting, Facebooking, emailing, and web surfing have pushed bedtimes ever later for all ages. I've been too tempted to stop and surf the web while reading on my iPad, so I've gone back to my Kindle for evening reading. Watching television provides just enough stimulation to stay awake and is tightly linked to obesity, so turn it off early!

The goal is to wind down gradually from your day. The *Atlantic* published a great article on how "Google makes us stupid," which asserted that the hundreds of web searches, texts, emails, tweets, and Facebook posts we do during the day fractionate our attention to such a degree that we no longer have any core knowledge. Reading long articles or books before bed allows you to slow down and integrate your knowledge into a bigger picture. You'll also calm your mind, which will help prepare you for sleep.

Establish a pattern. This is an important tip. For every hour that you sleep in on a weekend, your internal clock will take a full day to recover. So, if you get up at 7:00 A.M.

during the week and at 11:00 A.M. on Sundays, it'll be Thursday before you're back to normal. That makes for a pretty rough week! Set your alarm for the same time every morning, seven days a week. You may feel tired when the alarm sounds after a late night out, but, I promise, it's worth it. (Plus, you're probably used to the feeling due to this interesting little fact: We live on a planet with a twenty-four-hour day, but our internal clocks run on a twenty-five-hour cycle, so we always want an extra hour of sleep when we're young. As we age, our sleep-wake cycle shrinks to a twenty-three-hour day, which is why we begin to wake up early.)

Make your room a tomb. Don't use your bedroom for watching television, using the computer, or blasting music. Use window treatments that seal out the light and set the temperature to 68 degrees. Use white noise from a sound machine or fan to block out annoying sounds.

Get comfortable. A mattress chosen for your body type is crucial for sound sleep. The wrong mattress will cause back pain, wakefulness at night, and tiredness during the day, according to a Research Triangle Institute study conducted by Duke University sleep expert Andrew Krystal, MD. There is a new test you can take at mattress stores to select the appropriate firmness. The wrong firmness can allow your spine to bend in the wrong direction during the wee hours, when your spinal muscles finally relax completely.

Don't take your problems to bed. Examining every problem in your life will delay sleep for hours. Put them aside until morning. You can tackle any problem in the world if you wake up fresh, and you won't be fresh if you torture yourself while trying to go to sleep. Avoid arguments and heated conversations before bed as well.

Get good early-morning light. Your biological clock needs cues, and the best one to give it is a ray of morning light when you wake up. Open your drapes and look at the sky. If you wake in the dark, you can buy artificial lights that will simulate dawn anywhere in the world. During the dead of winter, program in a beautiful Brazilian sunrise. You'll be amazed at how it buoys your mood!

Pick a hotel chain and stick with it. I always try to stay at a Marriott hotel and have for years. They have the most consistent engineering that allows for a great night's sleep. The environmental units allow me to create white noise and cool the room down to 68 degrees, the perfect sleeping temperature. Their sheets, bedding, and blankets all feel like home.

Take your bedroom with you: I take a Tempur-Pedic pillow and eye mask with me everywhere I go so that I can make any place feel like home.

If you need convincing of the importance of sleep, consider this: Businesses lose $63 billion a year due to the underperformance of employees who've had a poor night's sleep, blowing big presentations and losing sales. More sobering, the National Highway Traffic Safety Administration estimates that drowsy driving "results in 1,550 deaths, 71,000 injuries and more than 100,000 accidents each year."[2]

EXERCISE: THE ULTIMATE TOOL IN WEIGHT CONTROL

People weren't meant to be sedentary. Hopefully you've already started exercising and are feeling its many benefits. In this chapter you'll find lots of great tips to help you kick your workouts up a notch if they're feeling stale. If you compete, we'll show you how nutrition can give you an extra edge.

"I exercise, but I don't see any results."

Two culprits are likely to be stalling your progress: faulty nutrition and inadequate exercise. Follow the recommendations here to make sure your efforts pay off.

Nutrition

FUEL UP

Make sure you have a protein-packed meal in the four-hour window before you work out. Veggies and lean poultry, fish, or black bean soup are prime choices. Do not load carbs just before workouts or races! Even if you weren't overweight before reading this book, you may have fallen victim to the hype about carb loading. Rather than fueling workouts as touted, carb loading pours a highly inflammatory load into the body. Gorging on pasta and bagels assaults every system, killing motivation and compromising workouts. Honestly, it's like being doped!

GO LOW CL

Reducing large spikes in your blood sugar will increase your energy, banish bonking, fatigue, and belly fat. Even very good endurance athletes carry spare tires around their middles that are vestiges of the old carb-loading tactic. Despite very intense training programs, too much bread and pasta goes directly to the belly and stays there. Slash your carb load and watch the spare tire finally vanish, while your endurance and pace climb steadily.

DON'T OVERLOAD

Don't reward yourself for a good workout with a 2,000-calorie dinner. Math is math. If you burn 300 calories exercising and eat 2,000, you're going to gain weight. Exercise does stimulate your appetite, so guard against it by drinking chia mixed with water or a sports drink during exercise and skip the reload unless you've done serious distance.

RELOADING

If you work out for an hour or longer, consider reloading afterward with a protein-carb sports drink specifically designed to refuel your muscles. In the 45-minute window after exercise your muscle cells are still open to the influx of sugar and protein. Reloading during this window prevents protein breakdown and can restock your muscle fuel stores for a great workout the next day. Pure Sport, a drink formulated for a study by John Ivy at the University of Texas in Austin, is a good choice for reloading.

Exercise Versus Activity

The public health community has long pandered to the American public on exercise, sending out the message that any type of activity is good. I have more faith in us, so I say: Don't be a wuss. You only live once. Put together a serious exercise program instead of just taking the stairs at work. (Taking the stairs will just get your work clothes sweaty and burn only a small handful of calories!)

Study after study has shown that activities such as gardening and manual labor lower the risk of everything bad: heart attack, stroke, sudden death, etc. It is fine to do these things as long as you realize that you are not burning many calories. All this activity may give you a ferocious appetite so you eat too much to take any weight off.

Vigorous aerobic exercise that employs many major muscle groups, on the other hand, is proven to aid weight loss. (Aztec activities, such as pulling 200-pound limestone rocks over dozens of miles or declaring war against the Spanish Empire, also burn calories but pose certain risks.)

Exercise That Burns Too Few Calories

We've already looked at the case of the big man on a recumbent bike, turning the cranks at a sleepy 40 RPM while slugging down a sports drink and talking to a pal for 20 minutes. There are plenty of other examples. The untrained swimmer, for instance, usually burns too few calories. Major muscle groups in the legs are underused, employed mainly to provide balance and flotation. In the Ironman, top swimmers cover a mile in 16 minutes. Most recreational swimmers take 30 to 60 minutes to swim a mile. Either ratchet up your training or choose a sport that will employ all the major muscle groups.

Intense Exercise

Once you're comfortable exercising, ask your doctor if you're okay to do more intense training. A very important recent study[3] of the morbidly obese showed terrific results after seven months of intense exercise and just moderate restriction of calories. The researchers found dramatic improvement in the following:

- Inflammation down 81 percent

- Weight down 39 percent

- Body fat down 65 percent

- Serum insulin down 52 percent

- HbA1 (hemoglobin alpha) down 11 percent

- Libido up 21 percent

Great for weight loss, intervals of intense exercise are also a highly effective training tool for more serious athletes. Intervals make you faster and increase your maximum VO_2 (oxygen consumption) and the stroke volume of your heart. They increase your speed and endurance, and they rip off the calories. Here's an example of an interval schedule for bike training. Within the course of a long ride, each interval should be done at the maximum intensity possible. I credit inspirational and legendary cyclist and coach David Wagener for this interval schedule. I use it religiously.

MONDAY: 16 intervals of 30 seconds each

TUESDAY: 10 intervals of 1 minute each

WEDNESDAY: 8 intervals of 2 minutes each

THURSDAY: 4 intervals of 4 minutes each

FRIDAY: 30 minutes at race pace

SATURDAY: Easy day

SUNDAY: Competition or hard ride

Vary Training Pace

The majority of amateur and weekend athletes do exactly the same workout every day with maddeningly little return. They'll run, bike, or swim the same distance at the same pace, which feels all-out but, in fact, is only about 70 percent of their potential. If you use the same intensity every day, you never fully recover, so you can't go fast. If you give yourself really hard days and really easy days, your strength, speed, and endurance will soar. Generally you want 48 hours between hard days, which may call for interval training or exercising at race pace. Take a day or two away from your primary activity and get on an Arc Trainer or other joint-friendly equipment. You'll see a drastic improvement in your performance.

"I compete and want nutrition to give me an edge."

This section is devoted to athletes engaged in endurance sports that burn vast amounts of calories over several hours, such as cycling, mountain biking, long-distance running, and hiking. The AD will let you train harder, faster, and longer than you ever have before.

Meal Planning

Make your workouts the ultimate priority in your meal planning. Breakfast sets the bar for the day. It's your best opportunity to load up on nutrients, especially antioxidants. Keep breakfast low in carb load so you won't have a blood sugar crash before you work out. For afternoon workouts, lunch is your fuel. This should be a combination of lean protein, veggies, and low-CL grains, consumed four hours before your workout so the food is digested and has moved from your stomach to your small intestine, where it will provide a steady supply of nutrients and keep your blood sugar level even. Eating a high carb load in the hour before exercise is the worst mistake you can make. After a fast rise in blood sugar, exercise will cause a rapid plummet, causing symptoms ranging from light-headedness to nausea.

Add antioxidants to your menu. As an athlete, you produce enormous amounts of free radicals that can damage your body and slow recovery dramatically. Eaten whole or in smoothies, antioxidants such as kale and cantaloupe will neutralize free radicals. Anti-inflammatory fruit and vegetable extracts can be added to your feed during long-distance events and to your recovery drink. Add quercetin or similar antioxidants to your supplement intake.

Before Your Workout

CHIA LOADING

A study from the University of Alabama at Auburn showed that chia loading[4] before long-distance events was as effective as carbohydrate loading. With the massive infusion of nutrients, chia loading far outdistanced carb loading on the antioxidant scale, speeding recovery. Chia is catching on quickly in the NFL too, reports the *Wall Street Journal*, among athletes who don't want to pump themselves full of supplements but still want to win . . . badly![5] I use chia before my weekly century cycling rides, putting three scoops into my breakfast smoothie that day.

CAFFEINE

Adding caffeine to a pre-exercise beverage[6] is a great way to burn more fat and improve your mood and your performance. Many studies, including a recent one from the Department of Kinesiology at CSU–San Marcos, confirm the finding of improved performance, showing a 2 percent increase in cycling performance in trained cyclists. I find that I always get a better workout with caffeine and would never race without it. Any form will do. I used NoDoz for my second Boston Marathon. I use Red Bull at the beginning of 100-mile events. Before routine workouts late in the day, I drink two cups of coffee during the morning. The effect holds over without my drinking caffeine in the afternoon, which would ruin sleep that night.

During Your Workout

Use fuels that improve your performance. Your muscles open up during exercise and suck in blood glucose without the need for insulin. This also means that you're not spiking your blood sugar during exercise if you drink beverages with higher amounts of glucose or maltodextrin. This is your chance to break the rules and drink beverages with higher carb loads. In the Tour de France, cyclists drink small Coca-Colas because they contain a mix of fructose and glucose. I drink them during my century rides. In long-distance competitions the problem is almost always too little fuel rather than too much. Here's the latest in fueling:

LAYERED SUGARS

The latest high-tech fuels are layered with different kinds of sugars, both glucose and fructose. Until recently the rule of thumb was 1 gram per kilogram of recovery sugars per hour for endurance events. That's roughly 60 grams of carbs per hour. A new British study[7] from the University of Birmingham, however, recommends increasing the new layered feeds to 1.5 grams per kilogram per hour, which can improve performance up to 8 percent. When ingested at a rate designed to saturate intestinal transport capabilities, drinks with added fructose or galactose were twice as effective as drinks with maltodextrin and glucose in replenishing liver glycogen during postexercise recovery, according to the university's research. The lead researcher, Dr. Asker Jeukendrup, found that a combination of glucose and fructose in a 2:1 ratio allowed endurance athletes to absorb and metabolize 50 percent more carbs every minute during exercise. Look for major sports drinks manufacturers to start reconstituting their beverages with this mix of ingredients. PowerBar C2MAX already incorporates this technology.

CHIA

New research at the North Carolina Research Campus conducted by Dr. David Nieman shows that during prolonged exercise the muscles preferentially burn omega-3 fats. Using a novel methodology called metabolomics, Dr. Nieman showed that all types of omega-3 fats including the alpha-linolenic fatty acids (ALA) found in chia seeds are taken from body fat stores and then burned as fuel by the leg muscles during running. To restore what is used during exercise, Dr. Nieman recommends an ALA-rich diet including nature's best source: chia seeds.

EXTRACTS

The harder you work, the more free radicals your body spews. Dr. David Nieman's lab has shown that the addition of antioxidants to exercise feeds improves recovery so athletes can go harder and farther the following day. Look for drinks such as FRS that contain fruit and vegetable extracts with powerful antioxidants.

PROTEIN

The use of protein in sports drinks was pioneered by Dr. John Ivy, who demonstrated that protein improves performance when consumed during exercise. The muscles can use the protein, as can the brain. He used in his studies a formulation called PureSport, which can be purchased online at www.puresport.com.

After Your Workout

REFUELING

Many people don't refuel after exercise because it seems counterproductive to ingest calories they've just worked to burn off. In fact, after prolonged exercise is the best time to refuel, because the nutrients consumed are used much more effectively by the body.

John Ivy's team found that individuals who consumed a CHO/PRO supplement postexercise lost more fat and gained more muscle than those who did not eat for two hours after exercise, although both groups did the same amount of exercise. A University of Birmingham study showed that carbohydrate consumed immediately after exercise goes directly into muscle fuel stores. This ability drops at least 50 percent after the first hour or so of recovery.

After exercise, the body enters a catabolic state in which it breaks down muscle protein if glycogen stores are not refueled. During this time you want to stimulate muscle protein synthesis and tissue repair, which enable adaptations in training.

What to drink? PureSport is a good choice. Gatorade also makes a recovery drink. Whatever you choose, look for a 2:1 ratio of protein to carbohydrate after strength workouts and a 4:1 ratio after endurance workouts. The combination of protein and carbohydrate elevates blood insulin and amino acid levels, which promotes glycogen storage and protein synthesis.

All of this means that recovery drinks will reduce soreness, prevent muscle loss, and speed rehydration. Aim to drink about half of the calories burned during your workout.

CHAPTER 12

THE URGE TO SPLURGE

Ugh! The pounds are creeping back on. The lure of french fries, croissants, burgers, pancakes, and bagels has proven too much to resist. You think you're doomed. But you are not! We all indulge ourselves. It's the easiest and most natural thing in the world to do. So, you ate a huge bowl of pasta, two pieces of bread, and a giant slab of tiramisu last night with three glasses of Chianti and a draft beer. Perhaps one monstrous meal led to a whole week of self-indulgence on your vacation. Don't worry! Now you can enjoy your splurges knowing that you can pull the extra weight off quickly and effectively by jumping back to chia smoothies for a few days. I do this after every trip instead of sweating about meals away from home.

One of the worst feelings for dieters is the sense of failure that comes with a big splurge. Keeping weight off is far more difficult than losing it, so difficult that the success rate is as slim as that for curing lung cancer: a meager 5 percent. The Aztec Diet is your solution to weight control. The premium foods and lifestyle changes we recommend will keep your weight down. When it spikes by a few pounds, there's no cause for panic—or resigned binge eating—because returning to a chia smoothie for breakfast will quickly turn the tide.

Furthermore, while a little food vacation may taste good, you'll probably find that the sudden exposure to highly inflammatory foods will make you feel so dreadful that you'll come running back to the AD, eager for clean, smooth energy and the satisfaction of watching those extra pounds fall away. So, don't fear giving in to the urge to splurge. Do it now and then. You'll find in time that you do it less and less. Here's the quick action plan for recovery:

RECOVERY PLAN

- Return to weighing yourself every morning.

- Return to Phase One, preparing chia smoothies three times a day.

- When you're within 2 pounds of your desired weight, return to Phase Two.

- When all the weight is off, return to Phase Three.

TROUBLESHOOTING

To help you hang on to your success, the AD gives you these methods to manage hunger at critical parts of the day and strategies for getting through special occasions that are notorious for derailing diets—without letting the weight you lost creep back on.

Managing Your Day

In the world of weight management, the two most important goals are kick-starting your day with the right breakfast and managing your night. Toward those ends, I opt to stay on a modified Phase Two pretty much all year. I have a chia smoothie for breakfast, a solid lunch, and a Gatorade with chia during my afternoon workout. Sometimes

I'll have a few handfuls of a healthy cereal in the evening, but that's often it for the night. This way I can take one or two nights out a week with friends, have a great dinner, and stay on track. If family dinner is part of your routine, be sure to choose AD meals and eat early!

EARLY MORNING

Weigh in first thing. Your weight may fluctuate as much as 5 pounds during a day, so having a consistent reference point is best. Use the bathroom before you weigh in. A pint of water weighs a pound, so you may get a head start right there. You'll also lose weight overnight, as respiration and transpiration through your skin eliminate about 2 pounds of water weight. If you had a big night out and you're up a couple of pounds, remember that you haven't actually gained 2 pounds; you just have that much digested food weight in your gut. If you stay on track for the next 24 hours, you can expect a big drop the next morning.

BEVERAGE PLAN

Start with tea or coffee. We recommend green tea for its smooth, swift energy boost. I use Ten Ren, a green tea that's imported from China, which I buy online once a year. It comes in a powder form that you can stir into cold water, making it totally portable.

Drink a glass of water before each meal. This helps to cut the calories you'll eat during the meal. Drink water with meals. Flavored beverages just add calories to your meal without affecting your satiety. Use caloric beverages instead as a treat between or after meals or during exercise.

BREAKFAST

The first way to prepare for a good breakfast is to eat well and early the night before. Waking up lean and hungry means you'll have a big appetite for great foods. Conversely, when you wake up after big, late-evening meals, you haven't slept well, you're not very hungry, and you crave things that seem light but carry high carb loads, like croissants and bagels. This is why the European breakfast consists almost entirely of white flour, jams, and butter.

If you're tempted to skip breakfast, don't. People feel virtuous when they skip breakfast, but then their blood sugar sinks and voracious overeating ensues. One poor food choice after another leads to thousands of extra calories. The National Weight Loss Registry shows that breakfast skippers unknowingly make up the calories they skipped at breakfast later in the day. "Eating a good breakfast is like putting gas in your car; it will provide you with the energy you need to start the day off right," says Roxanne Marshburn, a dietitian at Onslow Memorial Hospital. "One major misconception is that skipping breakfast leads to weight loss. In reality eating a healthy breakfast can help individuals with weight loss and with maintaining a healthy weight," she adds.

What you eat for breakfast is critical for setting up a successful day. Studies show that if you start your day with a low carb load you'll continue making low CL choices through lunch and even into the afternoon. The opposite is also true. When you start your day with foods packed with white flour: muffins, croissants, bagels, white toast, and the like you create hunger. The outpouring of insulin produced to confront a rapid rise in blood sugar creates hunger, which intensifies when the blood sugar crashes. This cycle creates a feeling of chronic fatigue and leaves you ravenous, poised to consume much more than you would if you'd set up your day properly.

A chia smoothie is the best choice for breakfast because it is low CL, delivers a lasting fullness, and energizes you with micronutrients. Put it in a travel cup or bottle and take it with you, drinking it gradually so it lasts a couple of hours. If you're not keen on the smoothie for breakfast, choose a meal from the menu in Chapter 9, like an egg white frittata or breakfast burrito. If you work out in the morning, mix a scoop or two of chia into a low-calorie sports drink or water to drink during your workout.

MIDMORNING

Have a big glass of water midmorning and another about an hour before lunch. If you had a chia smoothie for breakfast, you probably won't get the munchies. By lunchtime you'll have only a modest appetite, which will allow you to make good choices.

LUNCH

Start with a piece of lean protein and add some terrific veggies. Whether you make lunch or eat out, choose from the AD foods that are low CL and high in protein and omega-3s. Avoid disastrous high-carb lunches such as pasta and bread. They'll load you with calories and leave you dopey for the afternoon.

MIDAFTERNOON

Midafternoon is usually the first crisis point. We start to feel bored and fidgety. Our mood sours and we look for a quick fix—sweets or fast-burning carbs! These quickly turn into serotonin in the brain, which provides a soothing sensation. Serotonin is at a legitimate low here, and you do need to fix it. The best solution is to preempt the 3:00 to 4:00 P.M. blues with a good carb. At 2:30 or 3:00 P.M., have a mini chia smoothie or microwave half of a sweet potato, one of the world's healthiest, best-tasting veggies. The carbs will get into your system more slowly, but you'll be ahead of the blahs.

Another good solution if it's an option is a quick siesta. Recent research shows that a nap works better than caffeine at giving you productivity in the afternoon. You don't need much; sleep experts say that just 15 minutes of sleep has enormous restorative powers. Arianna Huffington set up nap stations at AOL when she moved in, and productivity soared!

REWARDS

The AD has built in a series of rewards so you have something to look forward to every few hours. Some rewards are pure pleasure; others are motivational. When you need something sweet, keep the portions small and try gum, colas, or chocolate.

LATE AFTERNOON

Late afternoon is the best time for a workout, just as you knock off the job. You'll be at your lowest mental ebb and your highest physical capability.

Your temperature, energy, motor coordination, thyroid, cortisol, sex hormones, and melatonin are all up by late afternoon, ready to fuel a great workout. (They're at a low at 6:00 A.M., which is why morning workouts are tough.) Warmer muscles provide more power, so you can train faster and longer in the afternoon. If you have absolutely no time at all, walk as far as you can after work. Park your car a few miles from work or take a bus, train, or subway a few stops farther away than you normally would, as this is the optimal time to burn calories.

DINNER

Contrary to popular custom, dinner should be the lightest meal of the day, not the heaviest. As the body burns less fuel while sleeping, food eaten late at night may be stored as fat, and digesting it can disrupt your sleep. Use the meals in Chapter 9 as guides until you're comfortable constructing your own high-protein, low-CL meals, and be sure to eat early. Try not to have more than 250 calories after 6:00 P.M. when you're trying to lose weight.

EVENING

Ground zero when it comes to dieting, evening is when most of us lose it. If your willpower is questionable, throw out or give away everything with high CL or fat content. Then do some defensive shopping. Stock your shelves only with the superfoods recommended in the AD, so if you have a fierce case of the munchies, nothing you eat will do terrible damage. A huge part of managing the evening is deciding what to do. Television is the worst choice as study after study links it to weight gain among kids and adults. If you must watch, go through some yoga postures while you do so. You'll avoid late-night eating and help wind down for bed.

BEDTIME

Go to bed hungry. You'll get a much better night's sleep and be ready to eat a healthy breakfast in the morning. You have to forgo the immediate reward of a junky snack, but you can train yourself to think instead of how great you'll feel the next morning.

EATING OUT AND SPECIAL OCCASIONS

Potential food disasters lie in wait for all of us, but a few good tips, a bag of chia, and a bit of willpower will keep you from grabbing for comfort foods or fancy treats and veering completely off course.

Cocktail Parties

I consider parties one of the worst challenges. You're stuck in a room for hours at a time. Alcohol fuels your appetite. Food is ever-present, wrapped in small calorie-packed morsels. Our strategy here is twofold: Immunize yourself by stirring 1 to 2 tablespoons of ground chia into a glass of cold water and drinking it before you go. Even if you are tempted by the hors d'oeuvres, you'll be pleasantly surprised at how few you eat. The next tip is to arrive late and leave early. This doesn't mean missing out on fun; think, instead, of distilling it. Be energetic, have good, spirited conversations, and leave when the inevitable lull settles, rather than staying for hours and leaving exhausted.

If you're the host and your guests are weight-conscious, consider that providing them with spectacular bacon-wrapped scallops, crabmeat, or an array of cheeses will make them feel awful and pay the next morning on the scale. Never do dieters feel more tense than when surrounded by a field of temptation! Serving healthier finger foods such as freshly cut fruit and veggies or bowls of edamame will make them feel great and be more at ease.

Restaurants

Often served in gigantic portions with shocking amounts of fat, calories, and sodium, restaurant meals can really sabotage you. The lack of nutritional information available, though it has improved in recent years, makes efficient eating tough, as you're basically ordering blind. Immunize yourself first with a scoop of chia and again, go for Japanese or fresh Mexican when possible. Stay away from Italian, Chinese, and steak houses. Skip the bread and go first for protein, which will fill you up and give you a natural stopping point. Remember the premium foods and order dishes that feature them!

You're probably too smart to fall for the lure of meals like the ones that follow, but seeing the magnitude of damage there will definitely help steel your resolve. In a 2011 article titled "Xtreme Eating," the food organization CSPI published a rundown of nutritional content in specific dishes at popular restaurants. Take a look at some highlights from this reporting and avoid this type of food like the plague:

- **THE CHEESECAKE FACTORY'S ULTIMATE RED VELVET CAKE CHEESECAKE:** 1,540 calories and 59 grams of saturated fat

- **IHOP'S MONSTER BACON 'N BEEF CHEESEBURGER:** 1,250 calories, 42 grams of fat and 1,590 milligrams of sodium

- **THE CHEESECAKE FACTORY'S FARMHOUSE CHEESEBURGER:** 1,530 calories and 36 grams of saturated fat with 3,210 milligrams of sodium

- **APPLEBEE'S PROVOLONE-STUFFED MEATBALLS WITH FETTUCCINE:** 1,520 calories and 43 grams of saturated fat with 3,700 milligrams of sodium

You *can* find healthy selections at these restaurants, just be discerning when you order.

Thanksgiving, Christmas, and Other Holidays

Holidays are like the Super Bowl of eating for most families. Perhaps the weather is cold and you've slacked off exercise. You're seeking comfort foods and facing a multiday celebration. The main event is a meal with enough calories to last an ordinary mortal a week. Even when it's not mealtime, you're likely stuck indoors. When the conversation runs out, boredom sets in; there is nothing to do but eat. You finally go to bed and find your entire sleep architecture disrupted. You toss and turn and burp till dawn.

If this doesn't sound so great, stick to the core concepts of the AD. First, get in a good walk or workout before the main holiday event. If you've been overeating, some of that fuel will end up as energy stores in your liver and muscles, which means you'll have added energy for a workout, so try to exercise longer and harder. Then drink two big glasses of water before you eat. At mealtime, avoid the high-carb foods such as mashed potatoes and dinner rolls. Fortunately, the main attraction at most holiday meals is turkey, which is the healthiest meat there is, so choose the white meat and eat plenty of it. For a sweet, filling treat, go for sweet potatoes. Even if you stray, remember that you have a flawless recovery program.

Weddings and Other Big Events

At times like these you're a sitting duck, exposed to thousand of extra calories and, let's admit, sometimes terrifying boredom. The toasts go on and on, and the best man's speech falls flat, leaving food as your best entertainment. Dinner lasts for hours, and you can't even order for yourself.

Again, immunize yourself with a stomach already full of chia. Go for the healthy hors d'oeuvres and dishes. You'll be pretty full from your chia inoculation, so even if you do splurge you won't be able to stuff in enough calories to do major damage. The next day, force yourself to get up at your normal rising time even if you feel dreadful.

Start the day with a chia smoothie even if you don't feel like having anything. This single step will put you right back on course, displacing the toxic food from the night before to get you feeling better fast.

Travel by Car

Drive-throughs spell death for a diet and, seriously, for many people too. When you're stuck in a car, there is no greater temptation than to pull off at one of the ubiquitous fast-food joints and load up with burgers, nuggets, fries, shakes, and colas. You don't even have to get out of the car! Quitting fast food will make drastic improvements in your health and weight. Put on your blinders and drive right by. Try to eat before you get in the car. If you've got a road trip to make, pack healthy snacks, or fill a thermos with a chia smoothie and sip it along the way to avoid temptation.

Travel by Plane

On a plane, you're trapped for hours in a narrow tube with your knees pinned to the back of someone's seat, and it's easy to use food as entertainment or consolation. In modern airports, the dazzling and tempting array of so many different kinds of foods can trigger major binges. This time chia can protect both your body and your wallet. Measure a few scoops into a plastic bag at home. Once past security, pour it into a bottle of water or gatorade and sip your way through the trip.

SUMMARY

There is one simple message, and it's this: DO have some of the foods you truly enjoy. DON'T eat out of boredom. You CAN recover with chia and the AD. When you step on the scales, you may be up 5 pounds or more after a single holiday or event. That's enough for many to give up hope. Don't. Just go back to your chia smoothie the next morning and at dinnertime. Have a great afternoon walk or workout. The following morning you may drop 3 or 4 pounds. Much of the extra weight you thought you were stuck with is what I call bowel weight. You have loaded your digestive system up with food bulk. If you've been smart and gone for the high-fiber dishes, there will be even more bulk. This will all start to wash out the next day. By the second day, you could be back at your normal weight.

APPENDIX

SYMPTOMS QUESTIONNAIRE

The following symptom survey will give a thorough picture of your health and any pain or discomfort you have, providing a great point of comparison for the improvements you'll feel on the Aztec Diet.

SYMPTOMS QUESTIONNAIRE: The following questionnaire was developed for you to track improvements in your mood, sleep, energy, and physical symptoms on the Aztec Diet.

INSTRUCTIONS: Before you start the Aztec Diet, fill in the first column, marked "Day 0." Every two weeks return to the table and enter how you feel.

SCORING: The scoring system is from zero to ten. Zero means the complete absence of that symptom. Ten indicates that the symptom is severe in its intensity. Mark your answer with a pencil in the columns below. If you have alarming symptoms such as shortness of breath with activity, tightness in the chest, or severe mood disturbances, review these with your doctor immediately. The most alarming symptoms are marked with an asterisk.

MOOD	DAY 0	DAY 15	DAY 30	DAY 45	DAY 60	GOAL
Anxious						
Depressed mood most of the day						
Difficulty concentrating						
Feel that everything is an effort						
Feeling blue						
Isolated						
Less interest or pleasure in activities						
Low confidence						
Low self-esteem						
Overwhelmed						
Poor self-image						
Relying on alcohol and sedatives						
Stopped doing things you enjoy						
Stressed by small events						

STOMACH	DAY 0	DAY 15	DAY 30	DAY 45	DAY 60	GOAL
Constipation						
Difficult or painful bowel movements						
Gas shortly after eating						
Heartburn						
Indigestion soon after meals						
Nervous stomach						

HUNGER	DAY 0	DAY 15	DAY 30	DAY 45	DAY 60	GOAL
Craving for snacks						
Always seem hungry						
Crave sweets in afternoons						
Eat when nervous						
Hungry between meals						
Excessive snacking at night						

SLEEP	DAY 0	DAY 15	DAY 30	DAY 45	DAY 60	GOAL
Difficulty returning to sleep after waking						
Difficulty falling asleep						
Difficulty staying asleep						
Early awakening						
Sleepy during the day						
Snoring						

ENERGY	DAY 0	DAY 15	DAY 30	DAY 45	DAY 60	GOAL
Fatigued						
Exhaustion—muscular and nervous						
Irritable and restless						
Reduced initiative						
Slow starter						
Tired all the time						

BODY	DAY 0	DAY 15	DAY 30	DAY 45	DAY 60	GOAL
Abnormal thirst*						
Afternoon headaches						
Back pain						
Can't cope with sudden increased activity*						
Feeling of "tightness" in chest*						
Headaches						
Heart palpitations*						
Hoarseness						
Increased sweating						
Joints ache on rising						
Joint pains						
Leg cramps at night						
Muscle pains						
Pulse fast at rest						
Sex drive reduced						
Shortness of breath with effort*						
Sneezing attacks						
Sugar in the urine*						

BLOOD WORK

Hopefully you had some routine blood work done before you started the Aztec Diet. Compare your results with these tables of normal values to see what kind of progress you need to make; then have the labs repeated after you've made it to Phase Three. You should see the numbers coming into line!

Cholesterol

These values should start to fall first in response to the Chia Challenge, in as little as five days. Large changes are seen after six weeks. These are the levels given by the American Heart Association.

HDL:

<40 mg/DL (men)	Major risk factor for heart disease
<50 mg/DL (women)	Major risk factor for heart disease
>60 mg/DL	Protective against heart disease

LDL:

<100 mg/DL	Optimal
100–129 mg/DL	Above optimal
130–159 mg/DL	Borderline high
160–189 mg/DL	High
>190 mg/DL	Very high

Triglycerides:

<150 mg/DL	Normal
150–199	Borderline high
200–499	High
>500	Very high

Fasting Blood Sugar

This test is the best way to tell if you're prediabetic. If your number is high, expect it to fall quickly. These are the numbers published by the NIH.

80	Healthy, no need for insulin or medication for diabetes
Below 100	Normal
100–125 mg/Dl	Prediabetes
>125	Diabetes (type II, adult onset)

Inflammation

Responsible for half of all heart disease and a host of other illnesses, inflammation makes people feel terrible.

CRP[1] (C-reactive protein. This takes a longer, more concerted effort to drop.) These are the results for the HS-CRP, which is the ultrasensitive C-reactive Protein Blood[2]

- Less than 1.0 mg/L = Low Risk for CVD

- 1.0–2.9 mg/L = Intermediate Risk for CVD

- Greater than 3.0 mg/L-High Risk for CVD

A1C A long-term marker of blood sugar control, this test is optional unless you have diabetes.

- Normal: Less than 5.7%

- Prediabetes: 5.7–6.4%

- Diabetes: 6.5% or higher

BUYERS' GUIDE FOR AZTEC GRAINS

Chia

Chia is available at health food stores, online, and from supermarkets like Whole Foods and Trader Joe's. I buy bags of microsliced chia and have them delivered to my home once a month. There is a vast range of quality out there, so find a good supplier and be willing to pay a bit more for better chia. Some cheaper brands have weeds mixed in with the chia, others are lacking in important nutrients.

The Aztecs discovered five hundred years ago that chia's power is unleashed only at a certain size and shape, so they learned to grind it. Less bioavailable, whole chia seeds don't work well in weight-loss studies. How the chia is ground is vitally important too. If the grind is too fine, the omega-3 fatty acids get squeezed out. If it's too coarse, the particles pass through the body without being absorbed. If commercially ground chia isn't cold-pressed, many of the phytochemicals and antioxidants may be destroyed, and it will go bad quickly. If you buy whole seeds and grind them yourself, eat them within a few days before they spoil. Unlike flax, chia seeds are very tiny and very hard to grind, so I recommend buying ground or microsliced seeds.

Look for seeds from Guatemala, Bolivia, Argentina, and Australia, regions that grow premium chia. Each strain has its own strength; some are high in fiber, others higher in protein, still others high in omega-3s. Look for chia that combines these premium strains in a blend.

Mila is a proprietary blend of chia from various regions in the world that is micro-sliced to increase bioavailability. It was used in our weight-loss study and exceeds USDA chia values by as much as 41 percent. Mila is sold online in 16-ounce bags and bulk shipments.

http://www.fueledbymila.net/challenge.

Spectrum Essentials Ground Chia Seed is a cold-milled ground chia sold at Whole Foods Markets in 10-ounce bags.

The Chia Seed is a brand of whole seeds sold online in bulk in 1.5-pound bags. www.thechiaseed.com

Health Warrior is a brand of whole seeds sold online and in some Whole Foods Markets in 16-ounce bags.

www.store.healthwarrior.com

Generic whole chia seeds are sold in bulk by www.nuts.com and www.bulkfoods. com in 1-pound, 5-pound, and 25-pound packages.

Navitas Naturals is a brand of whole seeds sold online and in some health food stores in 16-ounce bags.

www.navitasnaturals.com

Amaranth

Amaranth is a great, low-CL replacement for rice, potatoes, pasta, couscous, and oatmeal. Tough to find at regular grocery stores, amaranth is sold at most health food stores and through many online sites. Whole Foods Markets carry an amaranth hot cereal.

www.nuts.com/Organic_Amaranth

SUPPLEMENTS

Note: Always consult with your doctor before beginning a new supplement regimen.

SAMe

A chemical compound found naturally in the body and recently available as a nutritional supplement, SAMe (S-adenosyl-methionine) is used to treat osteoarthritis, bursitis, tendonitis, joint pain and inflammation, liver disease, migraine headaches, and other ailments. It's also said to have antiaging properties and to boost intellectual performance.

A recent study by ConsumerLab.com found that 30 percent of SAMe supplements selected for review failed their quality tests, so be careful in choosing a brand. Those that performed well include CVS, Doctors Best, and GNC, which are sold in 200- and 400-milligram doses. Look for enteric-coated tablets sold in blister packs (the brands just listed are sold this way), as SAMe degrades easily when in contact with heat or moisture.

Quercetin

During exercise the body produces damaging free radicals. Quercetin is a flavonoid antioxidant found in plants and vegetables that helps inhibit enzymes involved in free-radical production. It can be used to prevent and alleviate oxidative stress.

Dr. David Nieman tells us the best food sources of quercetin are onions, peppers, apples, and berries. Q Force is a quercetin supplement designed by the U.S. Defense Advanced Research Projects Agency to increase alertness, strengthen immune systems, provide energy, and reduce oxidative stress and muscle soreness after exercise. www.qforce.com

Fish Oil

Be careful not to overdose on fish oil if you're taking supplements, as more than 3 grams a day may increase the risk of bleeding. The amounts of EPA and DHA in products vary greatly. Look for 60 percent more EPA than DHA for its effect on mood. A recent ConsumerLab test showed quality problems with seven out of twenty-four products selected for review. ConsumerLab.com is a terrific resource on all supplements.

Glucosamine Chondroitin

If you're carrying a lot of extra weight, chances are good that your joints are strained. I believe that GC helps. I take 1,500 mg of glucosamine and 1,200 mg of chondroitin each morning to help repair cartilage in my joints. GC is a safer way to control joint pain than ibuprofen or over-the-counter medications that contain acetaminophen.

ACKNOWLEDGMENTS

I'd like to make the following acknowledgments:

HALEY NOLDE has put herculean effort into improving and organizing this manuscript. Haley is an incredibly gifted writer with a staggering ability to write clearly and cleanly. She has made this book both inspirational and fun. Haley lives in Richmond, Virginia, with her husband and three children. For fifteen years she's written for newspapers, magazines, books, blogs, and websites. Haley's passion for putting words on paper; her enthusiasm for feeding her family fresh, healthy, whole foods; her love of running, swimming, yoga, and pretty much any athletic endeavor made her a perfect partner for this project.

LISA SHARKEY has created more literary stars than Oprah. As producer on GMA and now senior vice president and director of creative development at Harper-Collins, Lisa has an incredible gift for picking winning concepts and shepherding them into bestselling books. Lisa was a tremendous help in shaping and positioning the book. Her infectious enthusiasm and dedication carried the day.

AMY BENDELL was the book's day-to-day editor and resource. Amy was always fun, cheerful, and incredibly helpful. Amy's knowledge and stress-free approach to editing made the book great and the job highly enjoyable. Her insights and direction were invaluable.

ALAN MORELL, my loyal agent of many years, shepherded *The Aztec Diet* through the key New York publishers and found a welcome home for it at HarperCollins. Alan has an incredible knowledge of the book marketplace and was of enormous assistance throughout the process.

MARY CORPENING BARBER AND SARA CORPENING WHITEFORD crafted the smoothies in this book. They're both inspirational mothers and gifted recipe writers. They created the art of the smoothie. I'm incredibly grateful to them for putting me together with Haley and for their friendship and guidance.

WALTER WILLETT and his team at Harvard are the best nutrition scientists of their generation and have set a standard for many to come. I await Walter's newest papers as I would a new bestseller. His work on glucose load and inflammation inspired the key principles in this book.

DEAN ORNISH has been an inspiration to me and has brought great credibility to the fields of nutrition and disease prevention with both his imagination and his rigorous scientific method. His pioneering work on heart disease, obesity, and prostate cancer was years ahead of its time.

OLDWAYS Sara and Dunn Gifford put the traditional diet back on the map as a solution for many of the world's populations. I have followed their work for decades and have watched with excitement and enthusiasm as they designed each new food pyramid.

JIM AND SHERRI WEAR for introducing me to chia and changing my life. Jim and Sherri are two of the kindest, most honorable and generous people I've ever met.

SARAH TOLAND is my long and trusted *Men's Journal* editor. Sarah was of enormous benefit in the original design of the project, its scope and vision. Sarah was invaluable in designing the premium foods section and laboriously sifting through myriad databases to come up with the best.

DAN GREEN had been my trusted colleague and agent for nearly a dozen books. Dan has razor sharp instincts and was responsible for many of my bestselling books.

CHARLES GAINES I wrote my first book with Charles Gaines, *Sports Selection*. Charles taught me how to craft books. Not a chapter goes by that I don't think of Charles and what he taught me.

CHARLOTTE HARDWICK has a tremendous flair for designing incredibly healthy meals. A graduate of the Integrative Institute of Nutrition in New York City, Charlotte did a spectacular job creating the menus and recipes in this book. They're fresh, inspiring, and delicious.

TERRI SHINTANI Terri's Hawaiian Diet set the standard for reintroducing traditional diets to native populations. His Hawaiian Diet proved that traditional cuisines could help erase the scourge of obesity and diabetes.

LIZZIE AND BARRY HINCKLEY for being both incredible friends and for first introducing me to chia.

KIMMY EVERETT for being a tremendous friend, pushing me to adopt the entire chia lifestyle and pushing life to the max.

NOTES

CHAPTER 1

1. Rich Ungar, "Obesity Now Costs Americans More in Healthcare Costs Than Smoking," *Forbes*, April 30, 2012, www.forbes.com/sites/rickungar/2012/04/30/obesity-now-costs-americans-more-in-healthcare-costs-than-smoking.

CHAPTER 2

1. Endoscopic Interventions for Weight Loss Surgery James C. Ellsmere1, Christopher C. Thompson2, William R. Brugge3, Ram Chuttani4, David J. Desilets5, David W. Rattner3, Michael E. Tarnoff6 and Lee M. Kaplan3

2. V. Vuksan, A.L. Jenkins, A.G. Dias, A.S. Lee, E. Jovanovski, A.L. Rogovik, and A. Hanna, "Reduction in Postprandial Glucose Excursion and Prolongation of Satiety: Possible Explanation of the Long-Term Effects of Whole-Grain Salba (Salvia Hispanica L.)," *Eur J Clin Nutr.* 64, no. 4 (2010):436–8. Epub Jan. 20, 2010.

3. V. Vuksan, D. Whitham, J.L. Sievenpiper, A.L. Jenkins, A.L. Rogovik, R.P. Bazinet, E. Vidgen, and A. Hanna, *Diabetes Care* 30, no. 11 (2007):2804–10. Epub Aug. 8, 2007.

4. S.S. Hassellund, A. Flaa, S.E. Kjeldsen, I. Seljeflot, A. Karlsen, I. Erlund, M. Rostrup, "Effects of Anthocyanins on Cardiovascular Risk Factors and Inflammation in Pre-hypertensive Men: A Double-Blind Randomized Placebo-Controlled Crossover Study."

5. A. Cassidy, E.J. O'Reilly, C. Kay, L. Sampson, M. Franz, J.P. Forman, G. Curhan, E.B. Rimm, "Habitual Intake of Flavonoid Subclasses and Incident Hypertension in Adults," *American Journal of Clinical Nutrition* 93, no. 2 (2011):338–47. Epub Nov. 24, 2010.

CHAPTER 3

1. Published Nov. 25, 2011, in the *Journal of the American Dietetic Association,* the study included 123 overweight and obese women between the ages of 50 and 75. The participants were taking part in a larger study designed to help them lose weight, and to examine the effects of diet and exercise on breast cancer.

CHAPTER 4

1. V. Vuksan, D. Whitham, J.L. Sievenpiper, A.L. Jenkins, A.L. Rogovik, R.D. Bazinet, E. Vidgen, and A. Hanna, "Supplementation of Conventional Therapy with the Novel Grain Salba (*Salvia hispanica L.*) Improves Major and Emerging Cardiovascular Risk Factors in Type 2 Diabetes: Results of a Randomized Controlled Trial," *Diabetes Care* 30, no. 11 (2007):2804–10. Epub Aug. 8, 2007.

2. D. Mozaffarian, and J.H. Wu, "(Ω-3) Fatty Acids and Cardiovascular Health: Are Effects of EPA and DHA Shared or Complementary?" *Journal of Nutrition* 142, no. 3 (2012):614S–25S. Epub Jan. 25, 2012.

3. www.hsph.harvard.edu/nutritionsource/what-should-you-eat/omega-3-fat.

4. S. Nodari, M. Triggiani, A. Manerba, G. Milesi, and L. Dei Cas, "Effects of Supplementation with Polyunsaturated Fatty Acids in Patients with Heart Failure," *Intern Emerg Med* 6 Suppl, no. 1 (2011):37–44.

5. A. Cassidy, I. De Vivo, Y. Liu, J. Han, J. Prescott, D.J. Hunter, and E.B. Rimm, "Associations Between Diet, Lifestyle Factors, and Telomere Length in Women," *American Journal of Clinical Nutrition* 91, no. 5 (2010):1273–80. Epub Mar. 10, 2010.

6. T. Hortobágyi, C. Herring, W.J. Pories, P. Rider, and P. Devita, "Massive Weight Loss–Induced Mechanical Plasticity in Obese Gait," *Journal of Applied Physiology* 111, no. 5 (2011):1391–9. Epub Aug. 18, 2011.

CHAPTER 6

1. http://yourlife.usatoday.com/fitness-food/exercise/story/2011-08-30/Study-Jogging-beats-weight-lifting-for-losing-belly-fat/50190566/1.

CHAPTER 7

1. *Science* 6, 200, no. 4342 (May 12, 1978):611–617.

CHAPTER 8

1. D.E. Sellmeyer, K.L. Stone, A. Sebastian, S.R. Cummings, "A High Ratio of Dietary Animal to Vegetable Protein Increases the Rate of Bone Loss and the Risk of Fracture in Postmenopausal Women," *American Journal of Clinical Nutrition* 73, no. 1, (2001):118–22.

Marian T. Hannan, Katherine L. Tucker, Bess Dawson-Hughes, L. Adrienne Cupples, David T. Felson, and Douglas P. Kieli, "Effect of Dietary Protein on Bone Loss in Elderly Men and Women: The Framingham Osteoporosis Study," 15, no. 12 (2000):2504.

2. L. de Koning, T.T. Fung, X. Liao, S.E. Chiuve, E.B. Rimm, W.C. Willett, D. Spiegelman, and F.B. Hu, "Low-Carbohydrate Diet Scores and Risk of Type 2 Diabetes in Men," *American Journal of Clinical Nutrition* 93, no. 4 (2011):844–50. Epub Feb. 10, 2011.

3. http://www.sciencedaily.com/videos/2007/0404-weight_loss_weapon.htm

4. N.M. Wedick, A. Pan, A. Cassidy, E.B. Rimm, L. Sampson, B. Rosner, W. Willett, F.B. Hu, Q. Sun, and R.M. van Dam, "Dietary Flavonoid Intakes and Risk of Type 2 Diabetes in US Men and Women," *American Journal of Clinical Nutrition*.

5. D. Mozaffarian, R.N. Lemaitre, I.B. King, X. Song, D. Spiegelman, F.M. Sacks, E.B. Rimm, and D.S. Siscovick, "Circulating Long-Chain Ω-3 Fatty Acids and Incidence of Congestive Heart Failure in Older Adults: The Cardiovascular Health Study: A Cohort Study," *Annals of Internal Medicine* 155, no. 3 (2011):160–70.

6. M. Strøm, T.I. Halldorsson, E.L. Mortensen, C. Torp-Pedersen, and S.F. Olsen, "Fish, Ω-3 Fatty Acids, and Cardiovascular Diseases in Women of Reproductive Age: A Prospective Study in a Large National Cohort," *Hypertension* 59, no. 1 (2012):36–43. Epub Dec. 5, 2011.

7. F. Campbell, H.O. Dickinson, J.A. Critchley, G.A. Ford, and M. Bradburn, "A Systematic

Review of Fish-Oil Supplements for the Prevention and Treatment of Hypertension," www.ncbi
.nlm.nih.gov/pubmed/22345681. *Eur J Prev Cardiol.* Epub Jan. 30, 2012.

8. H. Tong, A.G. Rappold, D. Diaz-Sanchez, S.E. Steck, J. Berntsen, W.E. Cascio, R.B. Dev-
lin, and J.M. Samet, "Omega-3 Fatty Acid Supplementation Appears to Attenuate Particulate Air
Pollution Induced Cardiac Effects and Lipid Changes in Healthy Middle-Aged Adults," *Environmental Health Perspective*, Epub April 19, 2012.

9. J.H. Wu, R.N. Lemaitre, I.B. King, X. Song, F.M. Sacks, E.B. Rimm, S.R. Heckbert,
D.S. Siscovick, D. Mozaffarian, "Association of Plasma Phospholipid Long-Chain Ω-3 Fatty Acids with Incident Atrial Fibrillation in Older Adults: The Cardiovascular Health Study," *Circulation* 125, no. 9 (2012): 1084–93. Epub Jan. 26, 2012.

10. A.P. Simopoulos, "The Importance of the Ratio of Omega-6/Omega-3 Essential Fatty
Acids," *Biomed Pharmacother.* 56, no. 8 (2002):365–79.

11. Lawrence de Koning, Vasanti S. Malik, Mark D. Kellogg, Eric B. Rimm, Walter C. Willett, and Frank B. Hu, "Sweetened Beverage Consumption, Incident Coronary Heart Disease and
Biomarkers of Risk in Men," *Circulation* 10 (2012).

12. M.M. Murphy et al., "Drinking Flavored or Plain Milk Is Positively Associated with Nutrient Intake and Is Not Associated with Adverse Effects on Weight Status in U.S. Children and
Adolescents," *Journal of the American Dietetic Association* 108 (2008):631.

R. Novotny et al. "Dairy Intake Is Associated with Lower Body Fat and Soda Intake with
Greater Weight in Adolescent Girls," *Journal of Nutrition* 134 (2004):1905.

R.H. Striegel-Moore et al. "Correlates of Beverage Intake in Adolescent Girls: The National Heart, Lung, and Blood Institute Growth and Health Study." *Journal of Pediatrics* 148
(2006):183.

13. Lee Hooper, Colin Kay, Asmaa Abdelhamid, Paul A. Kroon, Jeffrey S. Cohn, Eric B.
Rimm, and Aedín Cassidy, "Effects of Chocolate, Cocoa, and Flavan-3-ols on Cardiovascular
Health: A Systematic Review and Meta-analysis of Randomized Trials."

CHAPTER 11

1. J.E. Gangwisch, D. Malaspina, B. Boden-Albala, and S.B. Heymsfield, "Inadequate Sleep as
a Risk Factor for Obesity: Analyses of the NHANES I," *Sleep* 28, no. 10 (2005):1289–96.

2. http://www.nhtsa.gov/people/injury/drowsy_driving1/Drowsy.html.

3. N. Ahmadi, S. Eshaghian, R. Huizenga, K. Sosnin, R. Ebrahimi, and R. Siegel, "Effects of
Intense Exercise and Moderate Caloric Restriction on Cardiovascular Risk Factors and Inflammation," *American Journal of Medicine* 124, no. 10 (2011):978–82. Epub Jul. 27, 2011.

4. T.G. Illian, J.C. Casey, and P.A. Bishop, "Omega-3 Chia Seed Loading as a Means of Carbohydrate Loading," *J Strength Cond Res.* 25, no. 1 (2011):61–5.

5. "The NFL's Top-Secret Seed: Baltimore Running Back Ray Rice Puts His Faith in Chia Seeds, a Training Tool of the Ancient Aztecs," *Wall Street Journal,* Jan. 12, 2012, p. x.

6. T.A. Astorino, T. Cottrell, A. Talhami Lozano, K. Aburto-Pratt, and J. Duhon, "Effect of Caffeine on RPE and Perceptions of Pain, Arousal, and Pleasure/Displeasure During a Cycling Time Trial in Endurance Trained and Active Men," *Physiol Behav*, Feb. 12, 2012.

7. February 2008 issue of *Medicine and Science in Sport and Exercise*

APPENDIX

1. http://my.clevelandclinic.org/heart/services/tests/labtests/crp.aspx.

2. www.nlm.nih.gov/medlineplus/ency/article/003640.htm.

INDEX

vitamin C, 21
Vitamix, 34, 55
Vuksan, Vladimir, 13

W

waist circumference, 62
waist measurement, 30
Wakea (Father Heaven), 12
walking, 62
water, 127
weddings, 233–34
weigh-ins, 28–29

weight loss: and Chia Challenge, 26; chia's effect on, 6, 7, 42; and exercise, 80–85; and food volume, 11; and micronutrients, 21; and moving on to Phase II, 64; plateaus in, 29, 31, 56, 64; responsible, 27; and variety, 69
weight management, 227–28
wheat, 92
White, Oreann, 54, 55

Whiteford, Sara Corpening, 34
Willett, Walter, 15, 120
Wurtman, Judith, 59

Y

youthful appearance, 63–64

Z

Zone diet, 99

RECIPES

tomato juice, in smoothies, 43

tuna: salad sandwich, 71; and white bean salad over bitter greens, 168

turkey: and bean wrap, 73; burgers, 158; meat loaf, 196; sandwich, 73

tzatziki sauce, 177

V

V8 juice, in smoothies, 43

vegetables: basic frittata—build your own, 207; black bean stew, 190; frittata muffins, 171; lentil soup, 163; no-dairy egg white frittata, 156; quick lentil soup, 203; red lentil soup with kale and collards, 147; seasonal, lemon roasted chicken with, 179; in smoothies, 44; and white beans in parchment with poached egg on top, 166

vinaigrettes: apple cider, 150; creamy coriander, 167; Dijon, 158; lemon cumin, 183; sesame, 208; strawberry balsamic, 204

W

walnut-crusted halibut and quinoa, baked, 183

walnut red pepper spread, 160

watercress: white bean and tuna salad over bitter greens, 168

watermelon aqua fresca, 41

wood-plank-cooked salmon, 188

Y

yogurt: chia muesli, 176; curried millet salad, 195; curried sauce, 187; Dr. Bob's kale blueberry smoothie, 35; jasmine peach lassi, 37; as smoothie base, 42; tzatziki sauce, 177

Z

zucchini, shaved, salad, 178